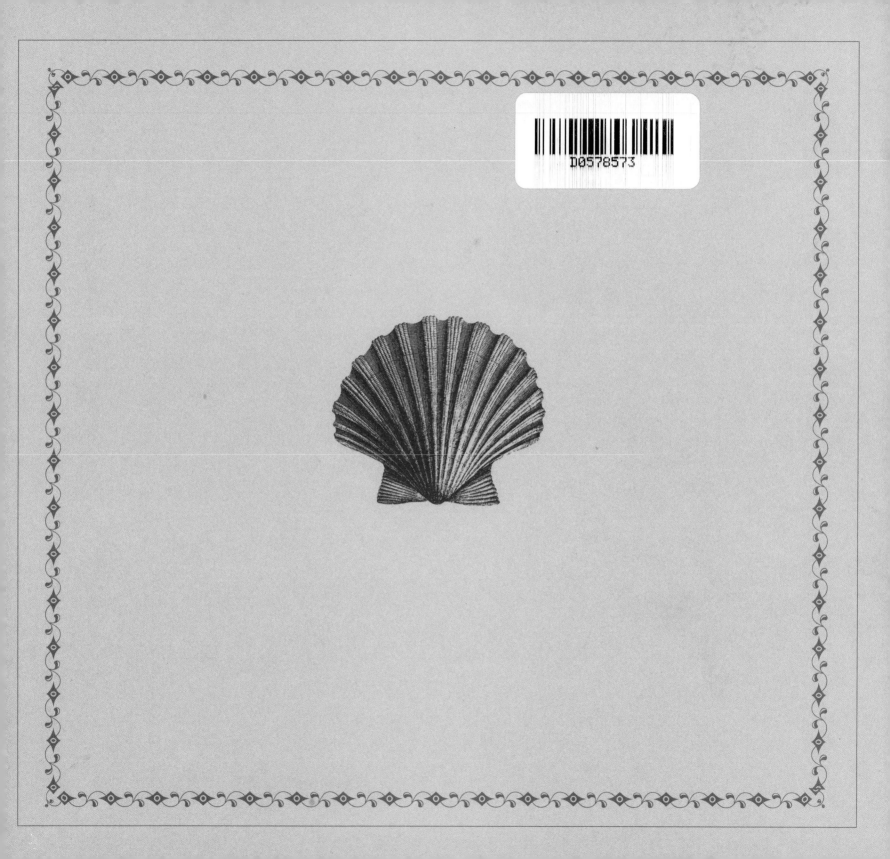

The
BATH AND BODY BOOK

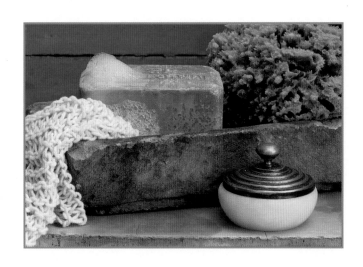

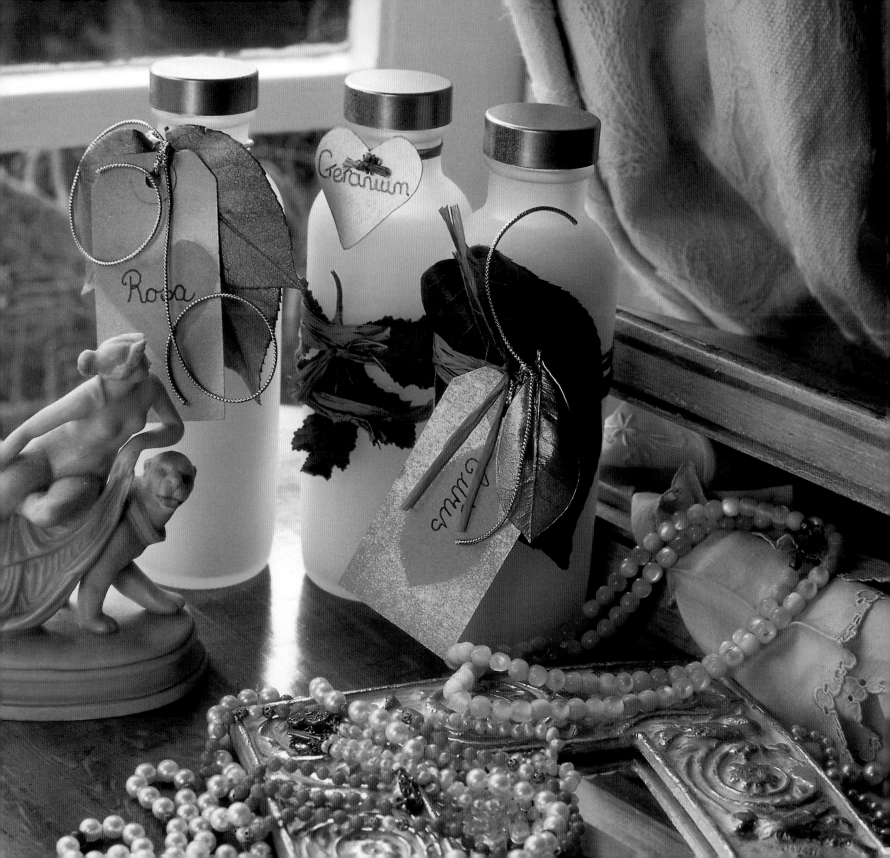

The BATH AND BODY BOOK

CREATING A PERSONAL OASIS WITH NATURAL FRAGRANCES,
SCENTED LOTIONS AND DECORATIVE EFFECTS

STEPHANIE DONALDSON

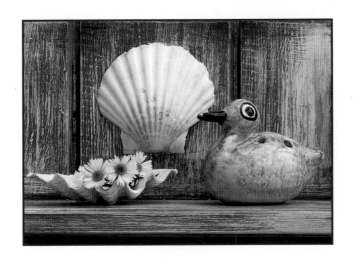

LORENZ BOOKS

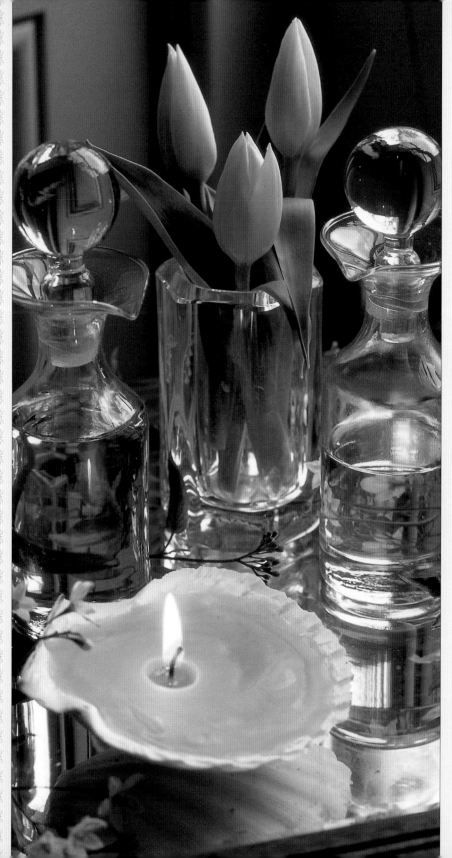

This edition first published in 1997 by Lorenz Books
27 West 20th Steet, New York, NY 10011

LORENZ BOOKS are available for bulk purchase for sales
promotion and for premium use. For details write or call the sales
director: Lorenz Books, 27 West 20th Street, New York,
NY 10011; (800) 354-9657.

ISBN 1 85967 391 0

Publisher: Joanna Lorenz
Project Editor: Joanne Rippin
Designer: Nigel Partridge
Stylist: Michelle Garrett

Printed and bound in Singapore

3 5 7 9 10 8 6 4 2

CONTENTS

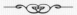

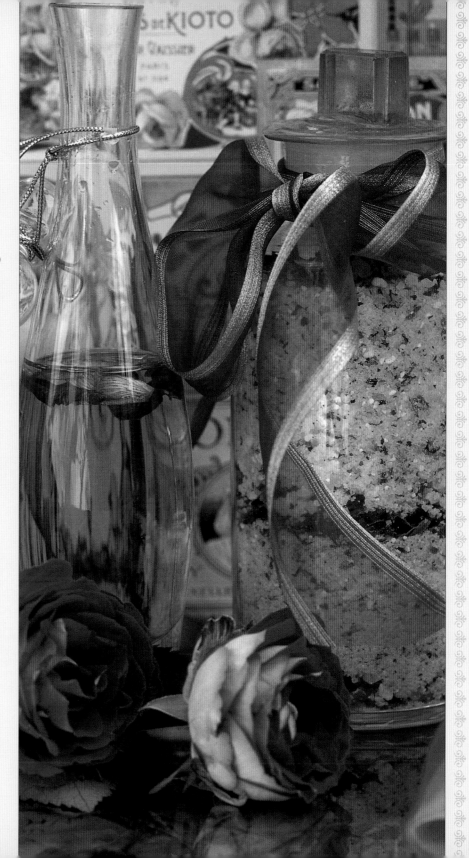

INTRODUCTION

"There is no place like a bath to stretch your soul and listen to your inner voice."
SENECA

*V*ery few of us own the bathroom of our dreams but we all own a bathroom in which we can dream. All that is needed to transform a bathroom into such a place is the decision to take the time to enjoy bathing, instead of viewing it as a task to be accomplished.

We generally live our lives at such a hectic pace that there is little time for contemplation or relaxation and we end up mentally over-stimulated and physically over-tired. In the middle of this hustle and bustle, we all need a refuge, a private sanctuary to which we can retreat and where we can put our own needs first, if only for half an hour. The bathroom can be this place and, although this book is partly about wonderful decorative projects and making luxurious lotions and potions, it is also about re-charging the batteries and taking time to care for the body.

Bathing is about so much more than cleanliness: it's about enjoying the ritual and discarding our worries along with our clothes, as we step into the warm water. The bath can be used as a place for creative thinking or a quiet reverie, as a comfort when life becomes unbearable or a place of permissible self-indulgence. Pampering our bodies with nourishing creams and lotions and using scented oils and colognes creates a feeling of well-being that we take into the rest of our lives as we emerge from the bathroom rested, refreshed and re-energized.

RIGHT: Choose ornaments, pots and bottles which complement your bathroom decor.

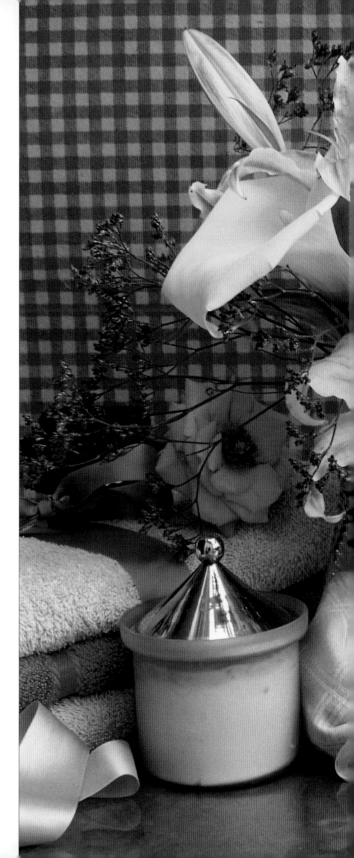

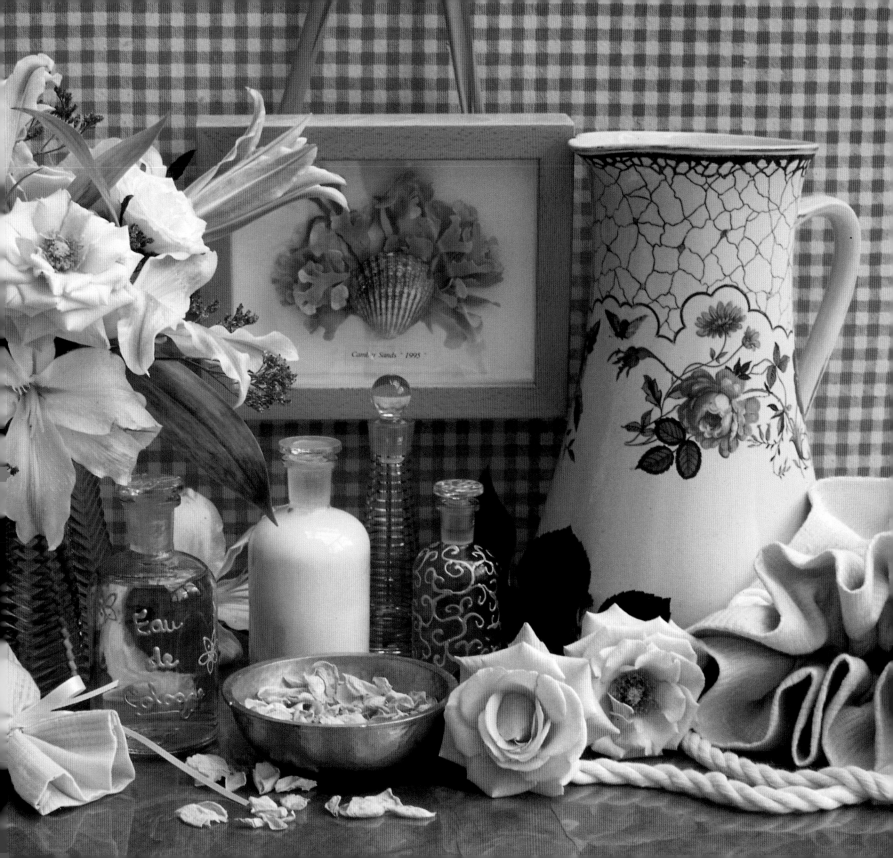

Camber Sands ' 1995 '

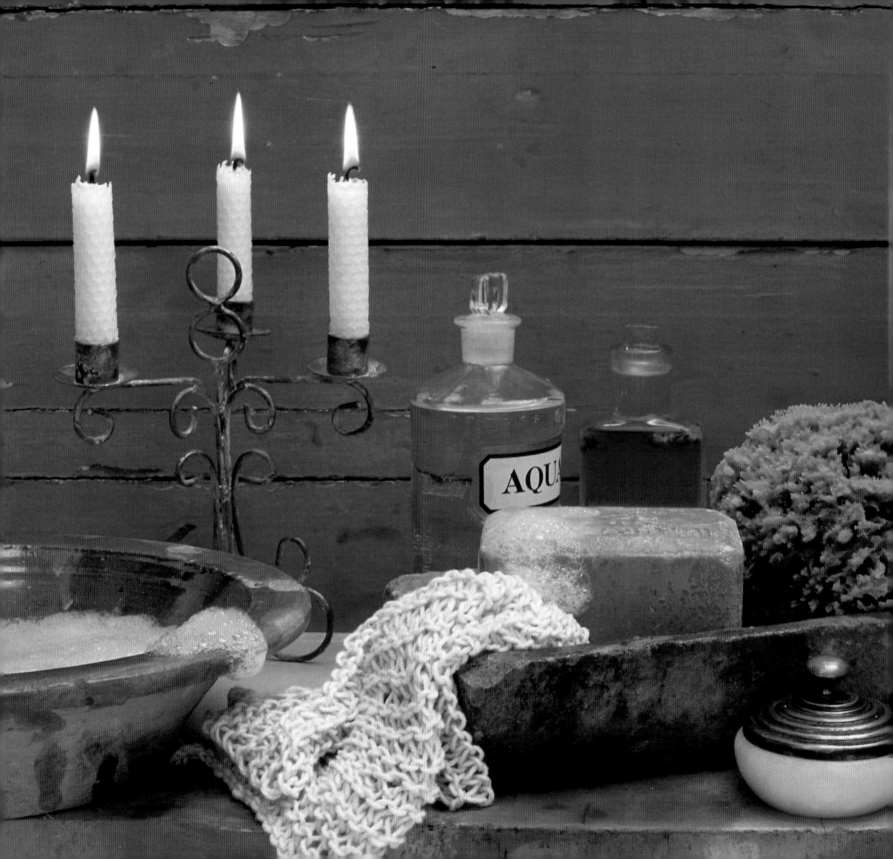

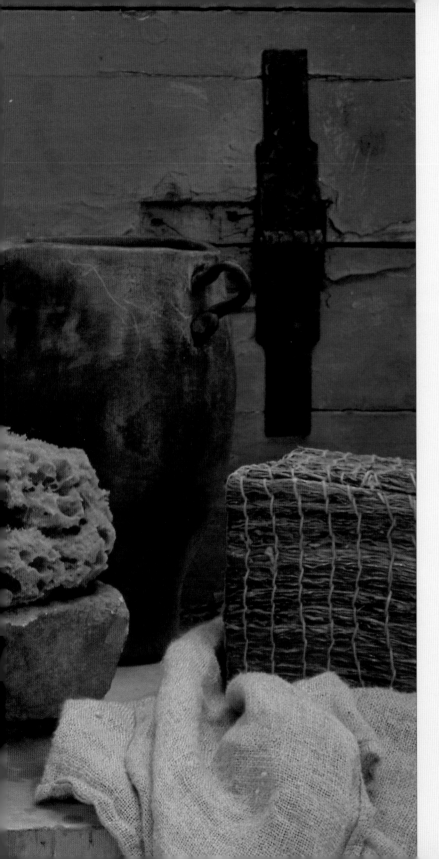

THE HISTORY
OF THE
BATHROOM

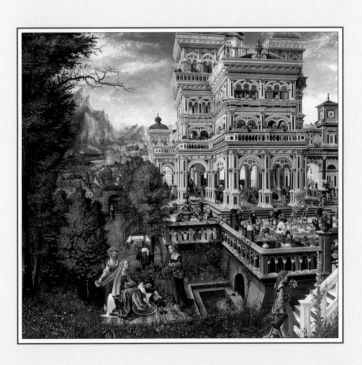

ABOVE: *A medieval lady is tended by her maids as she is bathed and groomed in a*

quiet garden away from the bustling activity which is taking place nearby.

LEFT: *The basic elements of our bathing habits through the centuries are timeless.*

BATHING THROUGH THE AGES

Ask schoolchildren what they know of ancient Rome and they will tell you that the Romans had baths with proper plumbing. This means far more to them than many of the other achievements of a great civilization and gives the past a reality they understand. It is the same for all of us: we may be awed by the great art and architecture which other civilizations have left but it is the experience of common humanity that helps us understand the people who have lived before us.

In earliest times, all bathing took place in natural springs and streams; with the advent of great civilizations came the ability to direct the flow of water to the cities and towns and

BELOW: Beautiful women disport themselves amongst the waves in an idealised version of bathing.

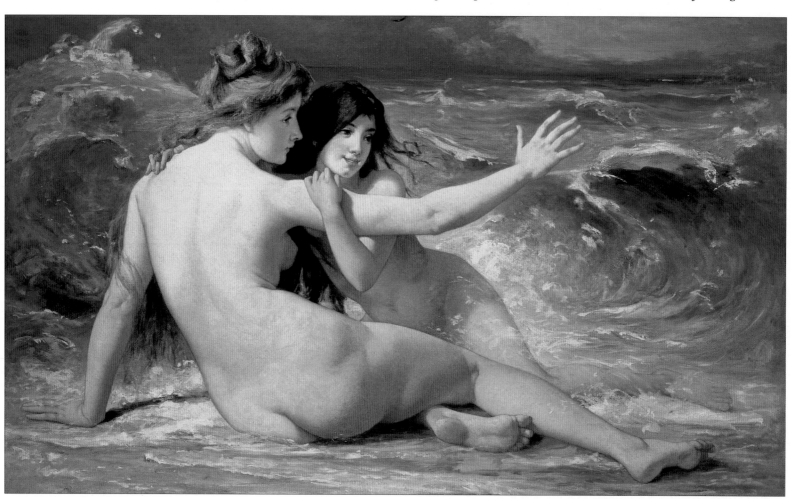

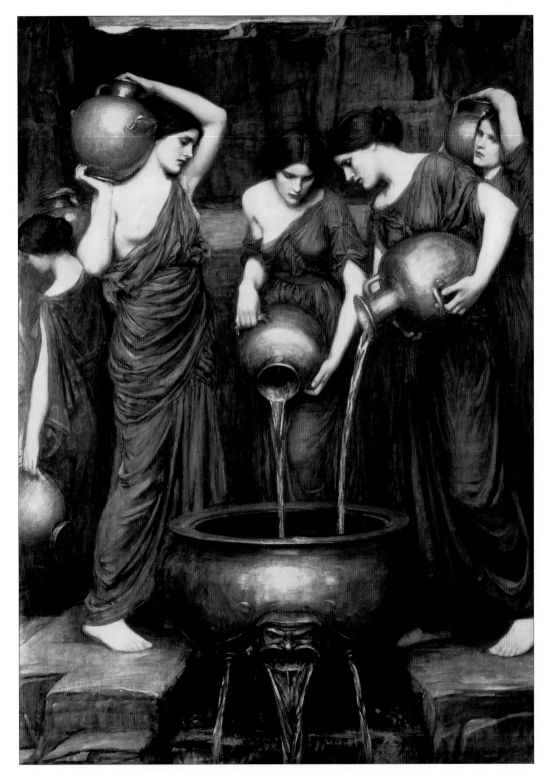

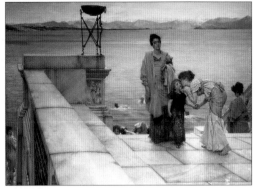

ABOVE: The Ancient Greeks were scrupulously clean and would bathe every day, generally in public.

LEFT: The water flows out of the copper bowl as fast as the maidens fill it, but many cultures viewed bathing in still water as very unhygienic.

incorporate pools and canals within their walls. There is evidence in Mesopotamia that irrigation works were carried out as long ago as 6000 BC and in the ruins of the Palace of Mari, built around 1800 BC, there is a bathroom with twin baths. It was not until the beginning of this century that personal bathrooms became available to most people; in the thousands of years that intervened, the use of communal baths for social and ritual purposes was central to most cultures.

The use of fragrant oils and perfumes has always been linked to bathing and they have a long history of being traded as precious commodities. Many fragrances, including myrrh, frankincense, cedar, cinnamon, saffron and spikenard were used in Biblical times as unguents and perfumes, and these and other herbs and spices from which these rare perfumes were made, were as precious as gold to the people of the Middle East at that time.

CLEOPATRA'S SECRETS

12 Many of the paintings and hieroglyphics of Ancient Egypt show the importance of bathing, both in religious ritual and in personal cleanliness. In the temples, priests were required to bathe in cold water four times daily, for purification, and their bodies were anointed with oils. During their religious rituals, the Egyptians burnt precious herbs as incense and it is likely that the hallucinogenic properties of plants such as marijuana were first discovered when they were used for this purpose. The priests were responsible for the making of fragrant oils, unguents and cosmetics and these were manufactured and stored within the temples. In the temple of Edfu, there are the remains of a storeroom for aromatics, whose walls were inscribed with recipes for many of the complex oils and perfumes that were made there.

All highly born Egyptians carried out elaborate bathing rituals, in baths scented with fragrant oils. They believed baths to be sensuous, calming and even religious. Baths were followed by massages with further aromatic oils, especially cedarwood oil, which was used to give the skin elasticity. There is a painting in one of the temples at Thebes that shows a high-ranking woman attended by her four servants, helping her with her daily adornment. Aromatic oils are poured over her body by two of the maids, while another massages her and the fourth holds a polished copper mirror in front of her.

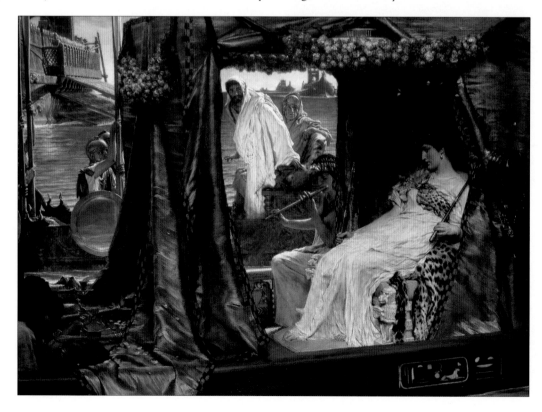

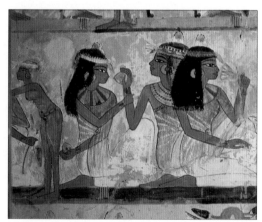

ABOVE: On the heads of the Egyptian women in this painting are perfumed wax cones which would slowly melt and drench the head and shoulders with perfume.

LEFT: Cleopatra awaits the arrival of the approaching Antony on her legendary perfumed barge which was made from fragrant cedarwood, with perfumed sails and hangings and decorated with roses, her favourite flower.

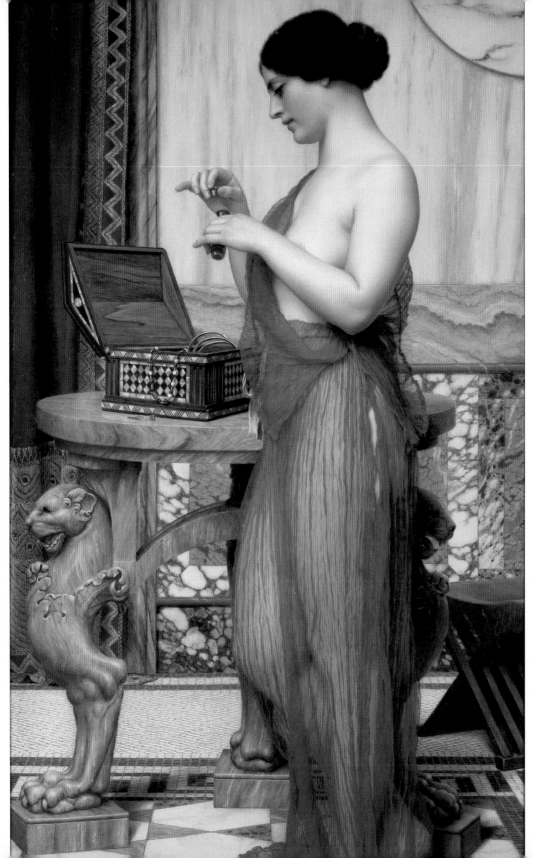

13

Cosmetics were considered to be essential and men also wore them for important occasions. Quince cream was used on the face and talcum powder, made from sandalwood, orris root and lemongrass, was used to scent the body. Kohl was used around the eyes and henna as a blusher, as well as to give the hair red highlights. The hair of the high-born woman was dressed with olive oil and elaborately coiffed. On special occasions, a wax cone of unguent would be held in position on top of the head by the hair. As the evening progressed it would slowly melt, covering the face and shoulders with a perfumed syrup.

Cleopatra, most famous of all the queens of Egypt, did not believe in the natural approach to beauty. She used every artifice to hand to make herself irresistibly alluring. Her use of fragrance was extravagant in the extreme and was not limited to her body: Antony had to wade knee-deep through rose petals to reach her bed and her ship was made of cedarwood, with sails made fragrant with cyprinum, her favourite perfume, made from henna flowers.

LEFT: Egyptian priests were experts in the making of perfumes and cosmetics and would supply these to high born men and women. Here a woman selects a perfume from a casket of bottles.

Nymphs and Naiads

*B*athing, predominantly for pleasure rather than as part of rituals, was important amongst the ancient Greeks, who would frequently take a cold shower before they dined. Pisistratus, who built many of Athens' finest buildings, also installed facilities for public bathing. Men and women bathed nude in public baths and showered in the cold water that spouted from stone ani-

BELOW: This Grecian vase shows a young woman at her toilette as she is attended by her handmaidens.

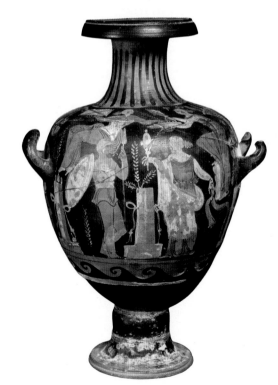

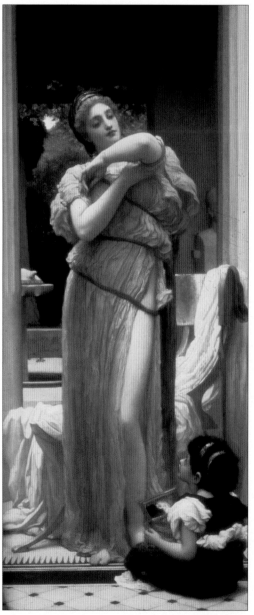

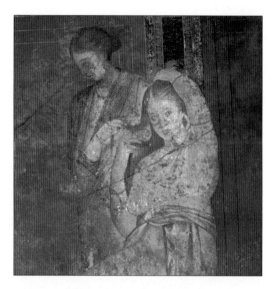

ABOVE: A delicate fresco from Pompeii shows a woman dressing her hair with the help of her maid.

LEFT: Like many little girls before and after her, this child watches as her mother completes her toilette.

mal heads. Ovid describes the beauty routine of a young Greek woman in the following words: "Her hair is smoothed with a comb; now she decks herself with rosemary; sometimes she wears white lilies; she washes her face twice daily in springs which trickle from the top of Pegasean woods; and twice she dips her body in the stream". Cleanliness indeed. Warm water was generally frowned upon as leading to indolence and weakness, although warm water heated in cauldrons was ladled over those who had excelled in battle and was also used to treat rheumatic pain.

Fragrant oils and unguents were used before and after bathing by the Greeks and much of their trade was based on their desire to obtain the materials to make these coveted cosmetics. The perfumes of Arabia were brought back to Greece by Alexander the Great and he also sent back many seeds and cuttings to the great botanist Theophrastus who wrote the earliest known treatise on scent called *Concerning Odours*.

RIGHT: The streets and squares of ancient Greece were filled with fountains and pools where the citizens would bathe in full public view.

BELOW: The pleasure the Ancient Greeks took in bathing is clear to see in this vase painting.

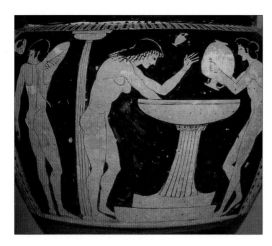

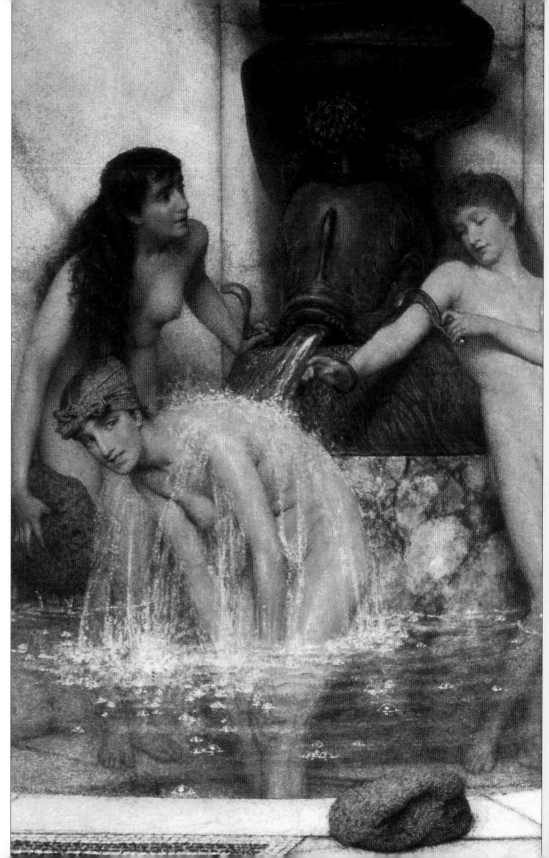

THE ROMAN BATHS

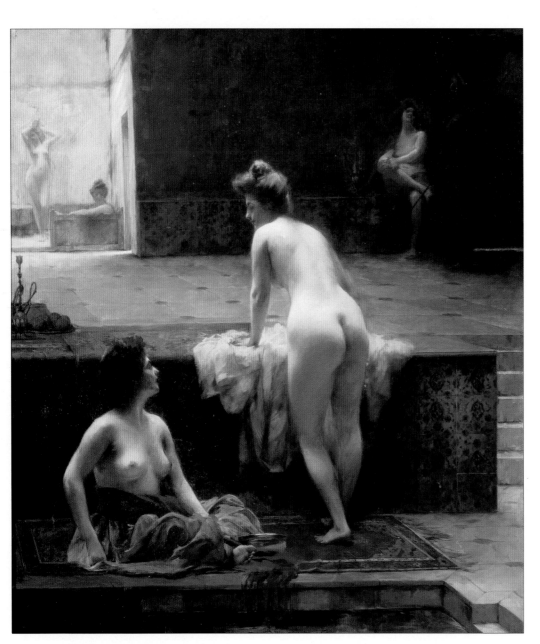

*I*n the early days of the Roman Empire, bathing was considered necessary but not particularly pleasurable. There was scorn for the hedonistic ways of the Greeks, and daily washing of hands and feet and weekly baths took place away from the light in gloomy, cramped rooms. The revolution was brought about by the introduction of the hypocaust, a system of underfloor heating of water and air. The Romans loved it and soon the new baths were at the centre of Roman social life. In vast public bath houses, they swam and exercised, exchanged gossip and enjoyed various fashionable therapies.

In the Caracalla Baths in Rome, 2000 bathers could be accommodated, each provided with a seat of polished marble. As the bathers arrived, they would hand their clothes to an attendant before first washing in cold water and then choosing from a range of options, including a massage, the swimming pool, the gymnasium, the steam room or a warm-water bath.

Cleansing the skin was generally achieved by scrubbing it with rough cloths, pumice or

LEFT: Roman baths were places of hedonistic comfort where bathing took place in beautiful surroundings.

RIGHT: Venus is pictured here at her bath as she is tended by Cupid and a handmaiden.

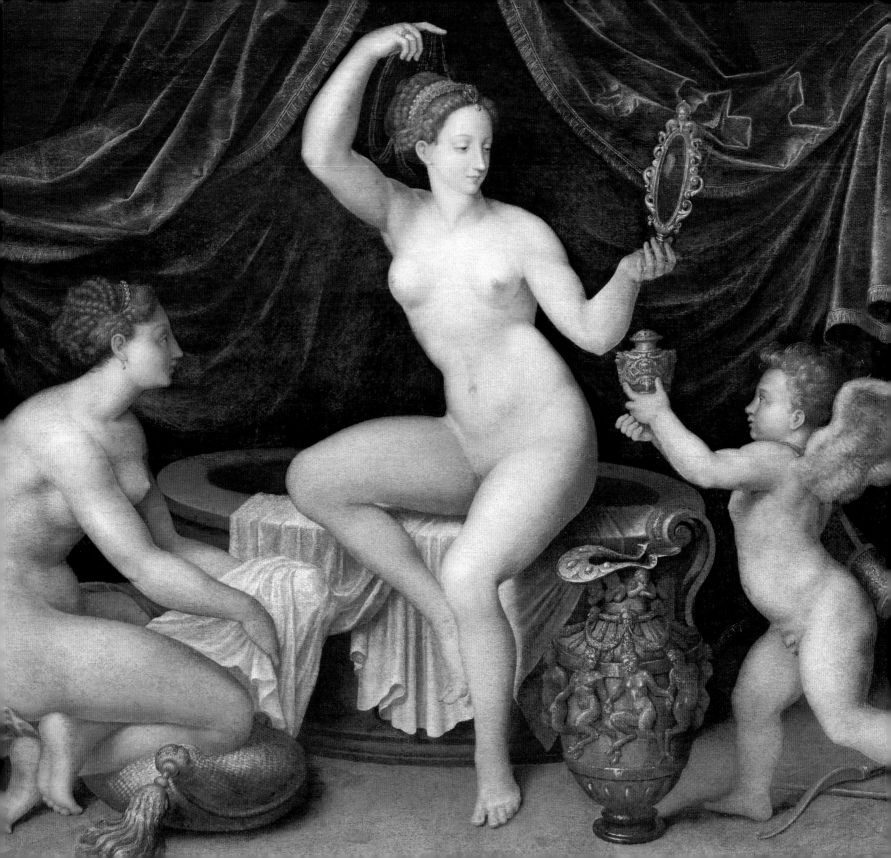

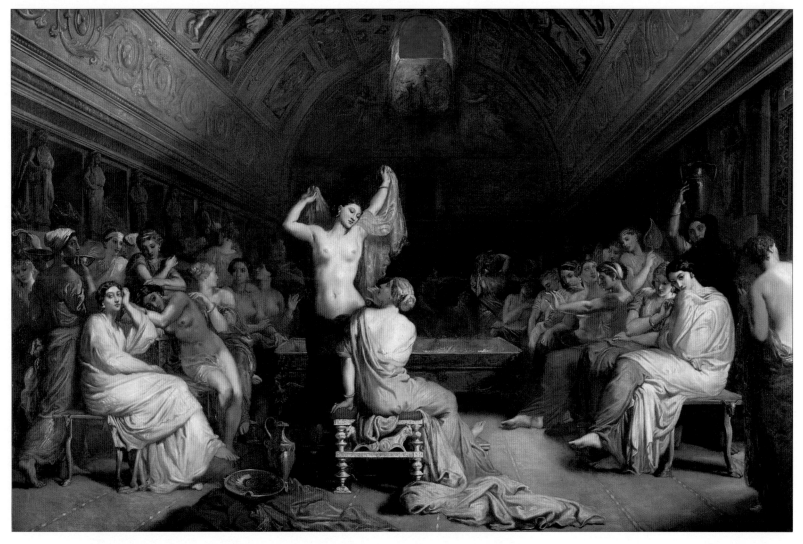

ABOVE: In Rome bathing was an important social event where news, gossip and confidences were exchanged.

clay, or by using a primitive version of the soap we use today, made from animal fat and potash. The word "soap" originates in a Roman legend, which tells how, after animal sacrifices on Mount Sapo (sapo is Latin for "soap"), the rain washed melted animal fats and wood ash down into the Tiber, where the scum that formed was found to be effective for washing clothing and skin. At the height of the Roman Empire there were 856 public baths in the city of Rome itself and, as the empire spread far beyond Italy, these magnificent buildings were built throughout Europe on such a grand scale that many of them survive to this day.

The Emperor Nero installed warm baths in his palace near the Colosseum and bathed in waters perfumed with rosemary and bay. Concealed pipes sprinkled fragrant waters on the emperor and his guests while they dined and ceilings painted like the sky would open and shower them with scented flowers – in such quantities that it is recorded that a guest was asphyxiated at one such revelry. The Romans were obsessed with roses: fountains were filled with rose-water, pillows stuffed with rose petals and they ate rose puddings.

With the decline of the Roman Empire, public bathing became less and less common throughout western Europe, with the exception of Iberia, where the Moors built hundreds of beautiful public baths as well as their magnificent palaces and gardens. When Crusaders from other European countries helped the Spanish to drive the Moors from Spain, they returned to their homes enthusiastic for continuing the warm baths they had learned to enjoy and bathing became a fashionable pastime amongst the nobility.

During the seventh and eighth centuries, there was a revival in public bathing and the Byzantines further developed the idea of steam-heating, which the Turks took over and developed when they conquered the Byzantine empire.

RIGHT: This painting of the famous Caracalla Baths shows their extraordinary opulence and scale.

BELOW: The faithful Penelope bathes Ulysses' feet. Footsore travellers were often ministered to in this way.

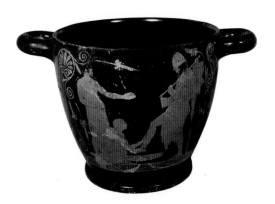

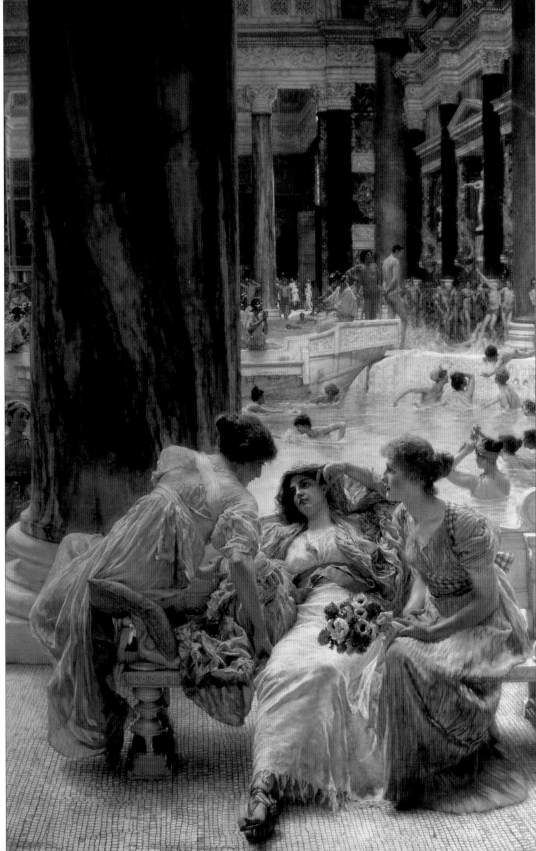

THE DECLINE OF THE BATH

Until the thirteenth century, bathing was the province of the nobility, who took weekly baths in their own homes. It became fashionable to entertain one's guests while bathing. The bath was enveloped in a draped cover and the bather and guests would listen to music, take part in flirtatious conversations and eat and drink elaborate confections while the bather soaked in scented water. It was around this time that public baths were once again established, although they bore little resemblance to the public baths of old. There

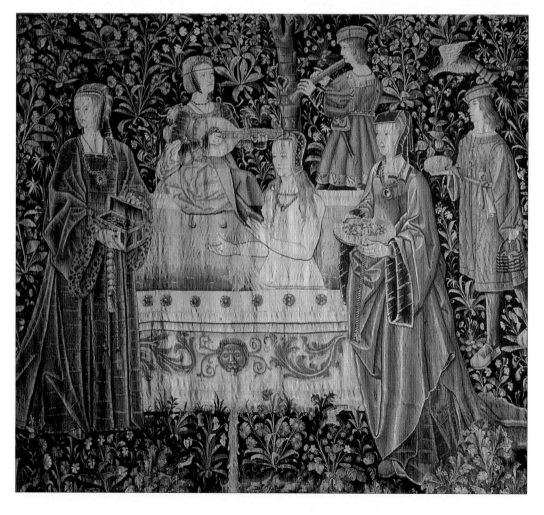

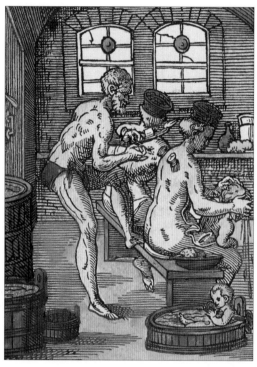

ABOVE: The communal bath house was a place where people could receive treatment such as "cupping".

LEFT: In the Middle Ages bathing was a social event amongst the nobility. Friends would attend and entertainment would be provided.

was no sophisticated plumbing and fresh running water; instead, water was heated in cauldrons and aromatic steam was produced by pouring herbal tinctures over hot bricks. While relaxing together, men and women could have their hair treated with herbal rinses,

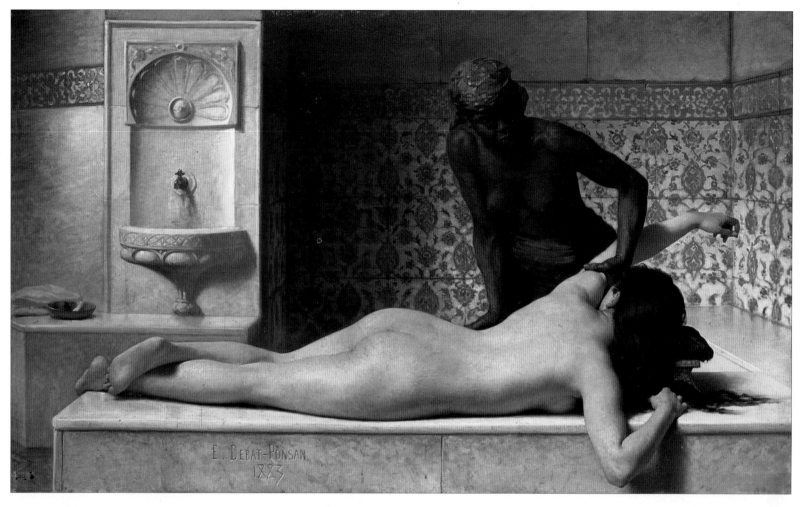

ABOVE: The spread of the Ottoman Empire popularised the Turkish bath with its attendant massages and other treatments.

LEFT: Communal bathing fell from favour in Europe when it was seen as debauched. It ceased altogether when science blamed the spread of the plague on water.

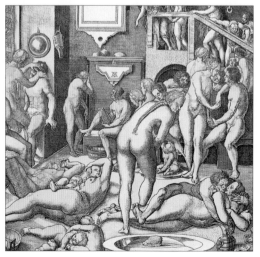

have a massage or undergo "cupping", which was a treatment for the relief of pain and involved placing heated cups on the skin.

The Church became more and more opposed to the public baths, convinced that they encouraged lewd and immoral behaviour, and, by the fifteenth century, few remained. These were finally closed as a result of the medical profession becoming convinced that water carried many diseases and, in particular, that infection with the plague could result from bathing.

This decline in public bathing facilities meant that for some time bathing was just not part of everyday life. From being thought of as a pleasure and a social occasion, washing was now seen as at best unneccessary, and at worst an unhygenic, even immoral activity.

A BATHLESS AGE

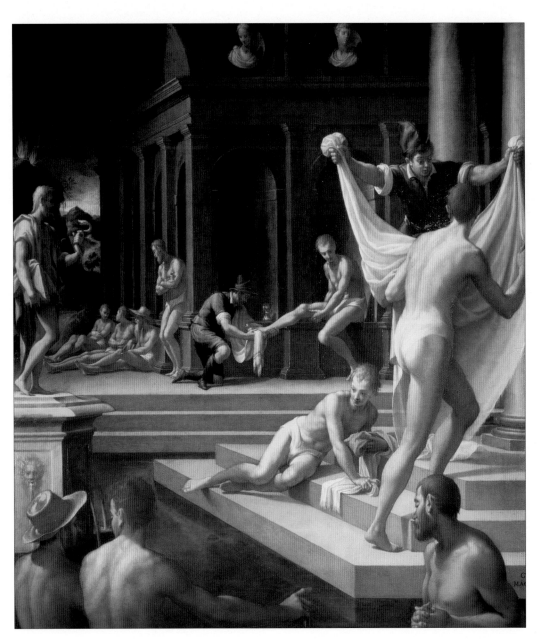

The fear of the harmful effects of bathing quickly spread across Europe, and in France the nobility soon became convinced that taking a bath could be fatal and they no longer used water for washing. Instead, they cleaned themselves with powders and used liberal quantities of perfume on their bodies and their clothes.

Louis XIV was known as the Perfumed King as well as the Sun King and he employed servants solely to scent his rooms and wash his shirts in fragrant waters. His Palace of Versailles was built without bathrooms, as was customary at the time, and, although six were added during his reign, they could not have made much impact in a building of 1300 rooms. It is recorded that he bathed only twice in his life and, on both occasions, became extremely ill as a result. He and his court concentrated instead on masking odours rather than washing them away.

Louis required a new fragrance to be created for him every day and he was much enamoured of table fountains, which shot jets of orange-flower water into the air. He also employed an idea first used by the Greeks and Romans and had doves drenched in perfume released at dinner parties, to scent the air.

LEFT: Bathing scenes of relaxed conviviality such as in the Pozzuoli Baths became increasingly rare in Europe.

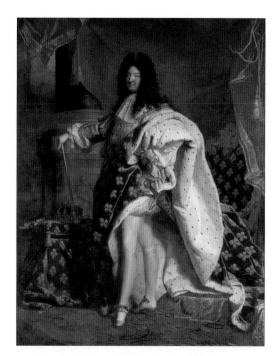

ABOVE: Louis the XIV, 'The Perfumed King', was recorded only to have bathed twice in his life.

RIGHT: Whilst Europe abandoned bathing, the Turks continued their tradition of rigorous cleanliness.

Britain, too, turned away from bathing and, in many ways, the Britons' approach to cleanliness and scent was somewhat less developed than that of their European neighbours. It was said of Henry IV of England that "he stank like carrion." Body odours were not always seen as unpleasant, though; "love apples" were made by a woman placing a peeled apple in her armpit until it had taken up her scent. She would then give it to her lover to remind him of his true love. Later the Puritans, who considered fragrances sinful, condemned the use of soap and water.

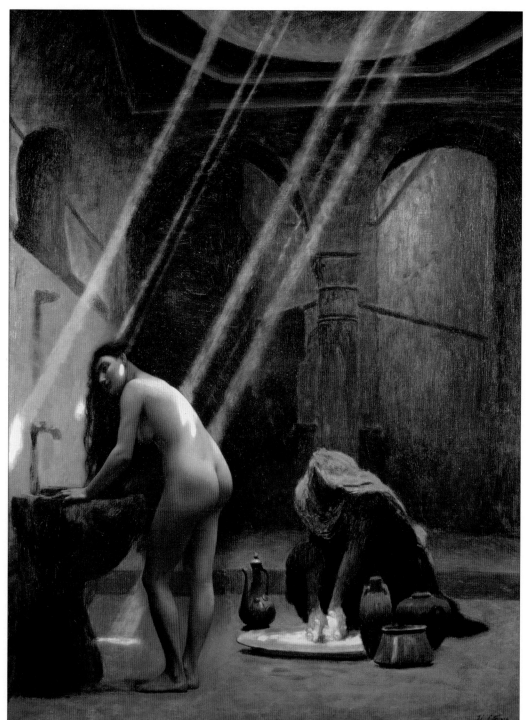

A REVOLUTION IN CLEANLINESS

24 It was the French Revolution that made bathing respectable once more and, indeed, fashionable. Under the influence of the fastidiously clean Napoleon, scientific knowledge became respected and the medical establishment began to see bathing as beneficial. An increasing number of public bath houses were opened and private bathrooms began to appear in the homes of the wealthy. As general hygiene improved, the soap industry became important. It was centred on Marseilles and the surrounding areas started to cultivate the aromatic ingredients with which the soaps were perfumed. Today, the olive-oil-based soaps of Marseilles are still widely used and have a reputation for quality throughout the world.

In complete contrast to their predecessors, doctors began to prescribe baths as treatments for many illnesses, especially bathing in the many spas and mineral baths, which were once again enjoying popularity. From the middle of the nineteenth century, regular visits to "take the waters" were considered essential, both for health and social standing. To be seen at the fashionable resort of the moment was of vital importance and the owners of these

BELOW: Under Napoleon's influence the French once again learned the pleasures of the bath.

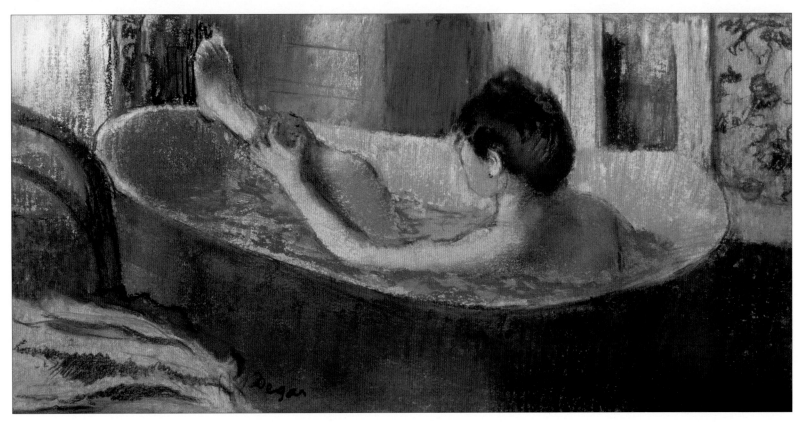

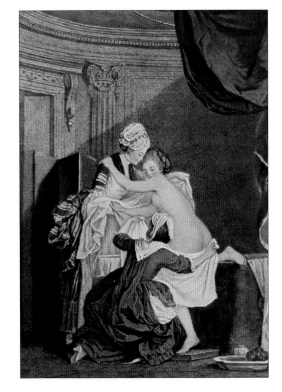

ABOVE: A lady of the sixteenth century is assisted from her bath by her maidservants.

RIGHT: In England, at the Pump Room at Bath, people of importance gathered to take the waters.

spas lavished huge sums of money on making the baths and their surroundings more and more luxurious. Towns that benefited from natural hot springs became wealthy from pandering to the needs of the rich and famous of society.

In the first half of the nineteenth century, water mains began to be installed in the major cities of Europe and in America and, with it, came the possibility of installing proper bathrooms in homes that had previously relied on

baths laboriously filled from jugs of water, which often had to be carried up several flights of stairs. Until the beginning of this century, it was still only the wealthy who could afford these luxuries but, for those who could, bathing was revolutionized. Inventors vied with one another to make more and more elaborate bathroom fittings, and tales of early water-heating systems make it clear that, on occasions, it would have required bravery as well as a desire for cleanliness to venture into the bathroom. Explosions and consequent fatalities were not unknown.

As running water was made available in the majority of homes, so bathroom fittings became simpler, more functional and a good deal cheaper. It became possible to install them in ordinary houses, where a small bedroom or the storage room was converted for the purpose, and new houses were designed and built with bathrooms. Many of these early bathrooms did not benefit from any form of heating, although some did have open fires, and it was not really until the advent of central heating that bathing for the general populace became the pleasure it is today.

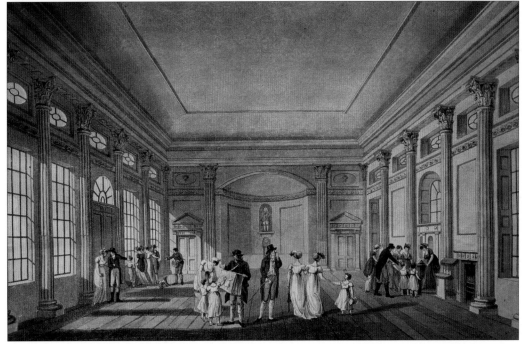

RITUAL CLEANSING

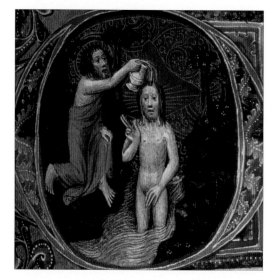

any of the world's great religions use ritual washing and bathing as important rites. It is seen as a symbol of spiritual purification and transformation as well as encouraging personal hygiene for health and well-being.

Within the Jewish faith, ritual bathing has retained its importance, especially in Orthodox households, and has changed little in 4000 years. Women are still required to be ritually cleansed after their periods and childbirth when they will visit a *mikwe*, a pool that is filled directly by a spring or rainwater.

Every religious observance or visit to the mosque within the Islamic faith must be preceded by a ritual cleansing, in which hands, arms, feet, face and head are washed in a prescribed order and manner in flowing water.

Although most Christian churches have reduced baptism to the symbolic marking of a cross on the child's forehead with water, the ceremony had its origins with St John the

ABOVE: The ritual purification of Christ by John the Baptist was given new meaning in the Christian religion.

LEFT: A painting of a Victorian family christening with the proud parents, their baby and the priest around the baptismal font.

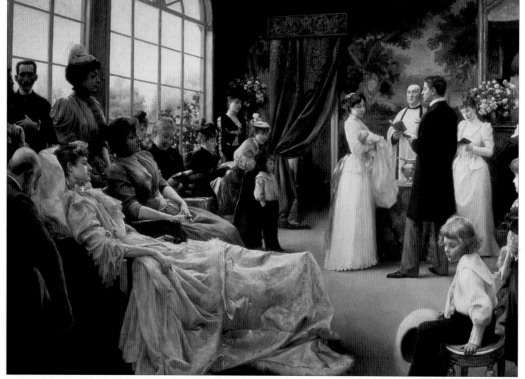

Baptist's immersion of his followers in the River Jordan, as a symbol of transformation, and some Christian denominations still practise baptism by full immersion.

In India, many religious rites centre on the sacred rivers, and bathing in these rivers is of great importance. When someone dies, the rest of the family bathes daily in a temple pool or river for eleven days, to release the spirit of the dead and bring calm to the family.

26

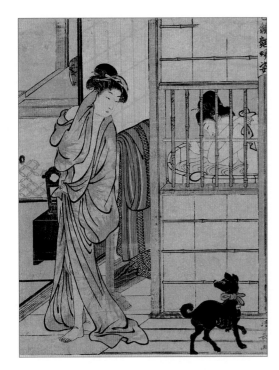

ABOVE: Japanese culture has always insisted on the highest degree of cleanliness.

RIGHT: The sacred rivers of India are central to most religious ceremonies and are used for ritual cleansing.

Native Americans have a long tradition of using hot springs for bathing and their sweat lodges are used for purification of the body and the spirit.

In Finland, saunas have been in use for 2000 years; they were originally earthen pits heated by hot stones. Women gave birth in them, ailments were treated and the dead were prepared for burial. Traditionally, the sexes were only mixed in a sauna within the family.

In Japan, public baths have been in existence since the beginnings of the Buddhist faith, with its emphasis on cleanliness to purify the body of sin and bring good luck. At a time when bathing in Europe was still recovering from disfavour, a traveller to Japan was astonished at the cleanliness of the Japanese, noting: "Everyone, no matter how poor, goes at least once a day to one of the public bathhouses that can be found in every town".

In Japan and China it has always been traditional to scent the environment rather than the body. It is interesting that in the people of south-east Asia the apocrine glands which create body odour are practically non-existent so there has been little need to mask unpleasant smells. In both countries incense burning was central to religious rituals based on the belief that the use of fragrance prolongs life.

The rituals of the bath are still observed in modern Japan, where it is traditional to wash oneself before entering the bath, which is seen as a place for quiet contemplation.

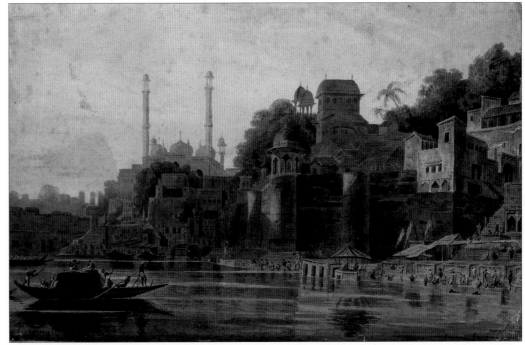

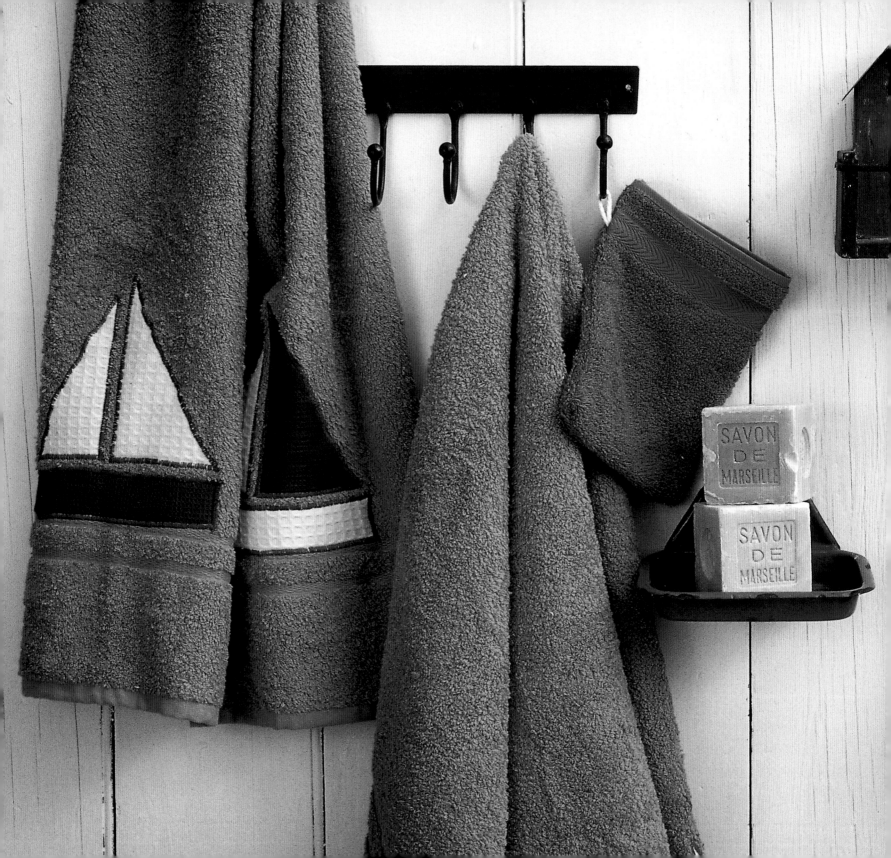

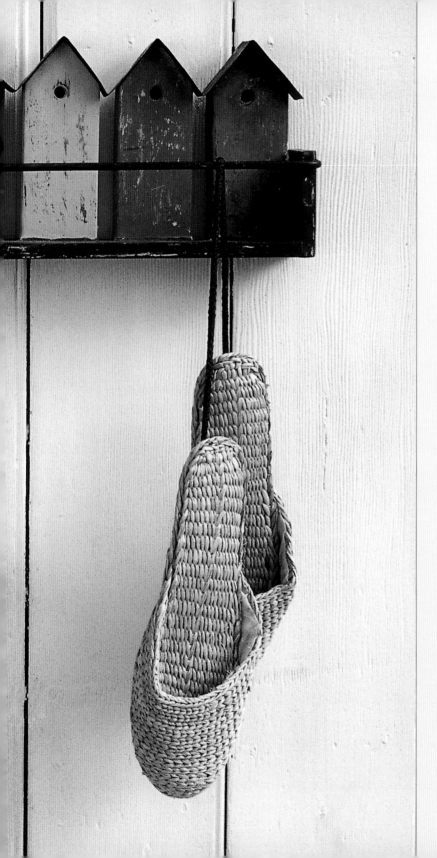

Chapter Two

THE
BATHROOM

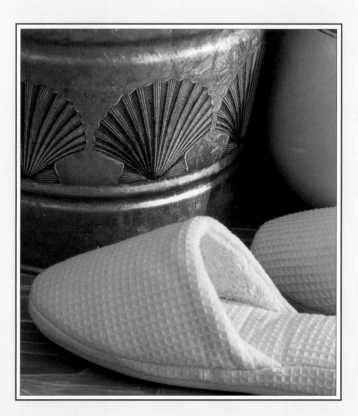

ABOVE AND LEFT: Decorate your bathroom so it becomes a welcoming haven

for quiet reflection and relaxation, rather than a last resort.

*I*t is a sad fact that most modern bath-rooms are small, functional and, frequently, uninspiring. Many builders and architects seem to think that we all long for a replica of a hotel bathroom: a windowless, fan-assisted, sterile laboratory that appears to have been crammed into a wardrobe at the furthest point from the window in the majority of hotel bedrooms. While it is true that, when we are away from home, our first priority is efficient plumbing and plenty of hot water, the home bathroom should be more, much more than that. It is a private refuge, a sanctuary where everyday concerns are soothed away in scented water and gentle self-indulgence is perfectly acceptable. For your bathroom to become such a place for you, it is important to make it a room where you are happy to linger, where your surroundings bring you pleasure and contentment and where company is an optional extra rather than an irritating interruption. To this end a lock, or hook on the door, is advisable. If necessary, this can be positioned high on the door to prevent children from locking themselves inside while they pour your precious bath oil down the drain!

RIGHT: This bathroom would do a Roman Emperor proud, the colours used are lovely and there are many elements which could be applied to a humbler bathroom.

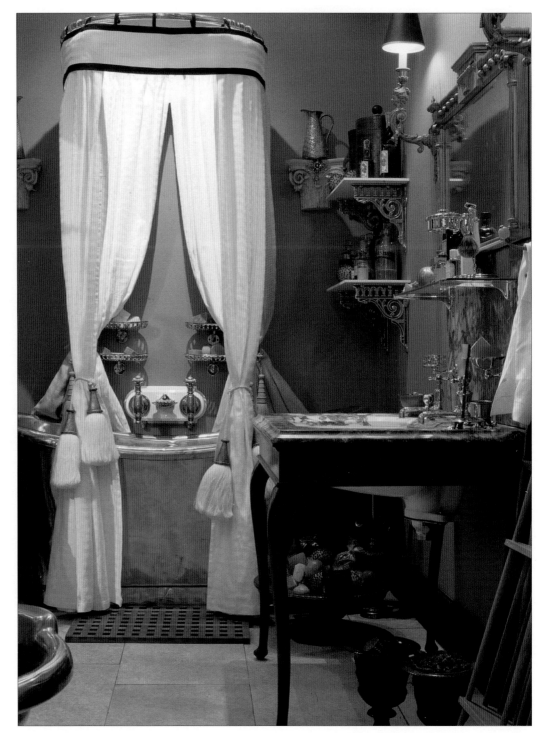

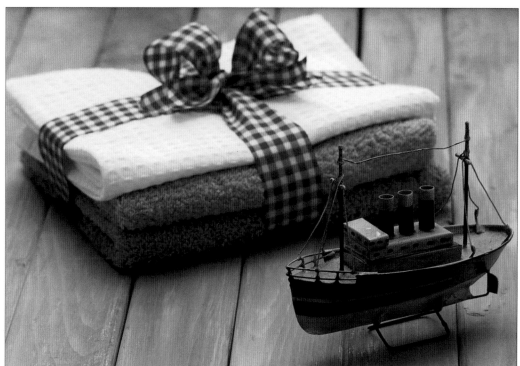

~ DECORATING ~

Decoration is a very personal matter but, in a small room, it is generally advisable to choose a single theme and build on it, rather than attempting to blend a number of styles, which will end up looking cluttered rather than co-ordinated.

Fortunately, the last twenty years have seen

BELOW: String bags are a great way of storing bits and pieces in the bathroom, especially anything which may get musty if not allowed to drain.

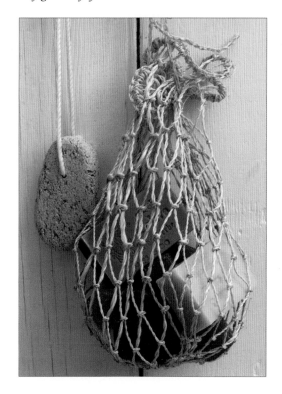

ABOVE: Towels tied with pretty bows become decorative as well as functional.

a return to predominantly white bathroom fittings, after a foray into pink, turquoise and avocado, and estate agents no longer boast proudly of "coloured bathroom suites" in their particulars. It is far easier to add colour and character to a neutral white bathroom than to transform a bathroom featuring an avocado suite and tiled to the ceiling with patterned beige and brown tiles (although,

even here the situation is far from hopeless and gutting the room is not the only option). Obviously, your budget is an important consideration but even those on a shoestring can bring about wonderful transformations with the application of tile paint and the purchase of some new towels.

It is not practical to attempt to paint a coloured bathroom suite and, if you really hate your suite, the only solution is to replace it; but it can be made much less dominant if you decorate the rest of the room in bold

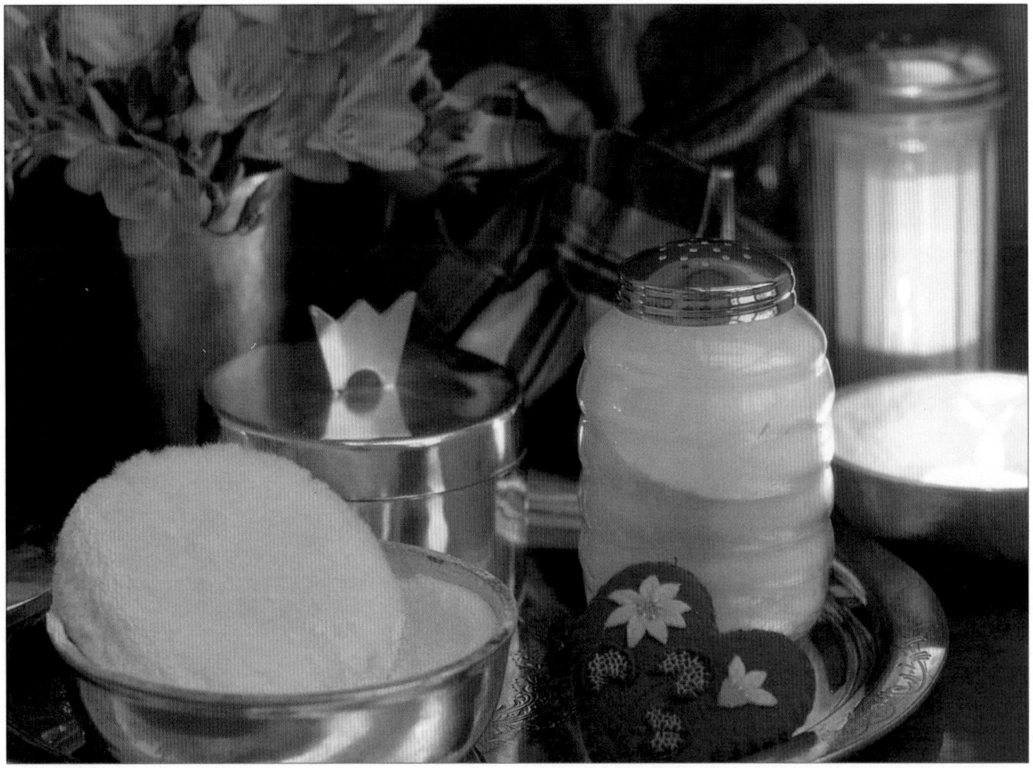

colours that draw the eye away from the offending fittings. Tile primer, an oil-based undercoat, is available from specialist paint manufacturers and can be applied to wall tiles, providing they are thoroughly cleaned beforehand. Once the undercoat has dried, a coat of gloss paint in the colour or colours of your choice will complete the disguise.

Although the finish will not be as perfect as a glazed tile, it is reasonably hard wearing and will cover a multitude of sins.

Above: Soft lighting in a bathroom is much prettier and more flattering than strong lighting.

LIGHTING

Lighting in the bathroom should be soft but practical. Rather than flooding the whole bathroom with light, an illuminated magnifying mirror is a good investment. This is useful for close inspection and allows the room to be more subtly lit than normal. At its simplest, this can be achieved by using one of the softly tinted light bulbs that are now readily available in many shades, including pink, peach or apricot, which are most flattering to the skin. The addition of candles or lanterns will provide a golden glow for moments of self-indulgence or romance.

HEATING

Efficient heating is essential in the bathroom and should, if possible, include an electric towel rail, which will dry towels when the heating is switched off. Damp towels are unpleasant to use and quickly start to smell.

FLOORING

The choice of flooring really depends upon who uses the bathroom regularly. Small children and carpets are seldom compatible. Wood, vinyl or linoleum are far more practical, with the addition of machine-washable cotton mats for warmth and comfort. Tiled bathroom floors are generally more popular in hot climates. In cool climates, they give an impression of chilliness in even the warmest bathroom and are very unforgiving if you fall. Growing children bring an amazing amount of debris into the bathroom – dried mud from the day-before-yesterday's sporting activity, sand from a visit to the beach and lawn trimmings – which manage to adhere to every layer of clothing. At this age, children are on the look-out for excuses to avoid cleanliness and being told off about messing up the bathroom provides them with ready ammunition. So, once again, go for a hard-wearing practical surface that will not cause unnecessary family conflict. Similarly, teenagers like to experiment with hair-dye, nail varnish and all manner of cosmetics which are not carpet-friendly.

For those whose bathroom is genuinely a personal oasis, not invaded by any of the aforementioned, such practicalities need not apply and carpet is the luxurious solution.

⊸ *PLANTS* ⊷

Wherever possible, plants should have a place in the bathroom, although this is obviously not practical in bathrooms without windows. Plants soften what is often a hard environment as well as adding colour and scent. Ferns are particularly happy in the damp atmosphere and will thrive in a bathroom where a shower regularly fills the air with droplets of moisture. Scented plants, such as jasmine, stephanotis or scented-leaved geraniums, do well on the bathroom windowsill; the leaves of the geranium can be crushed and dropped into a bath for added fragrance.

RIGHT: The natural-look bathroom uses a nice blend of natural materials and subtle colours.

⊸ *CHOOSING A STYLE* ⊷

There are certain styles which work particularly well in bathrooms of any scale and some of these are featured in the projects in this chapter. The "Natural Look" is a style that features natural materials, such as wood, shells and sponges, as accessories to subtle tones of white, cream and beige.

The addition of layers of the warmer tones of cream and beige, in paintwork, towels, flooring and fabric, softens the starkness of white and creates a subdued but sophisticated impression. At its simplest, by using tatami matting (a woven rush or bamboo matting from Japan) on the floor, a cream blind at the window and natural wood accessories, you can create your own version of a Japanese bath house. For those who find minimalism too

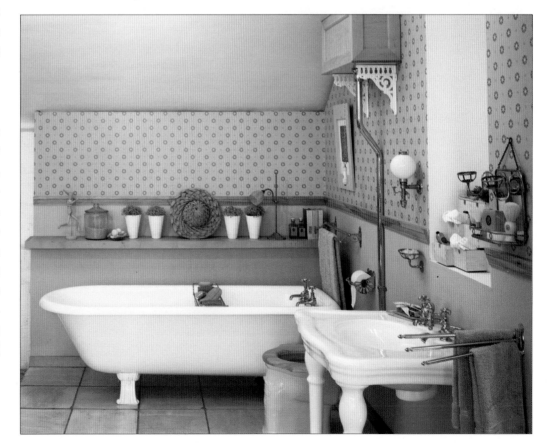

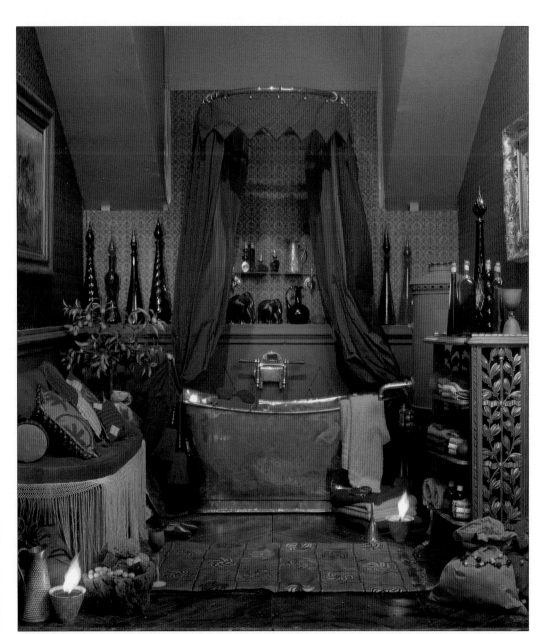

34

difficult to sustain or not sufficiently sybaritic, the addition of carpet, curtains and even a comfortable chair will create a more opulent effect, especially when lit by scented candles.

The "Classical Look" is an option for those who hanker after the luxuries of ancient Rome. The addition to a plain white bathroom of decorative motifs and accessories in bronze, gold and turquoise will soon create a luxurious impression.

Paint wooden or solid floors to resemble mosaic, marble or stone and varnish them, to ensure durability. It is fun to play with scale when using classical designs and, generally, it works best when the scale is large. A single urn painted a metre (3 feet) high on a blind will create more impact than several small ones. Pretend that your bathroom is a fragment of a far larger room and furnish and decorate it to that scale and you will create your own Roman Bath, with the promise of all the attendant pleasures.

The "Seaside Look" is perfect for a family bathroom, especially as the finish and appearance of weathered wood – much admired by designers – is ideal for surviving the heavy wear and tear children can inflict.

LEFT: This classic-look bathroom has Renaissance Italy meeting Byzantium. Deeply coloured walls and sumptuous hangings surround the copper bath.

There is no point in having a pristine bathroom filled with elegant accessories and precious perfumes if the reality of your life is that you have a boisterous family who splash water everywhere, use your perfume as a substitute deodorant and leave damp clothes on the deep-pile carpet. At least in a bathroom with a seaside theme you can pretend, when you finally evict everyone else, that you are floating in warm sea just off-shore from a desert island, or better still, a deserted island.

Once again, a white bathroom is a good starting point and, if you are starting from scratch, you have the option of lining the lower two-thirds of the walls with tongue-and-groove boarding, instead of tiles. A narrow shelf running around the top of the boarding is very useful for storage, especially in a small bathroom, and can also be used to display shells, toy boats and other seaside memorabilia. Plain white tiles can be stamped or stencilled with patterns of seashells, fish or boats and woodwork painted in a strong marine blue, sea green or white. Don't bother with carpet: use washable cotton rugs on a wooden floor that has been sanded and sealed, to avoid the risk of splinters. Towels in bright, seaside colours complete the theme.

If the "Seaside Look" is too vibrant for your taste but you like the appearance of distressed wood, the "Scandinavian Look" is a

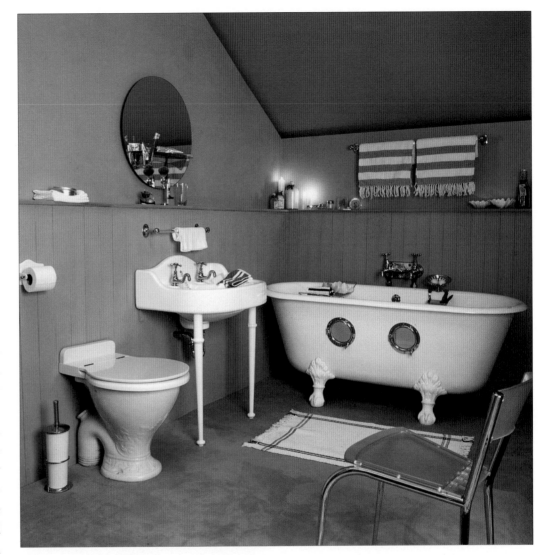

subtler alternative. Soft grey-greens and blue-greys are painted in layers on off-white or cream and rubbed back, to show the paler colour underneath. Simple stencil motifs can be used to add further decoration to the walls, while checked fabrics and towels in slightly deeper tones will add highlights. A floor painted to give the appearance of weathered boards would look great in this bathroom.

ABOVE: This seaside bathroom has incorporated a touch of quirky humour by the addition of portholes to the bath, while the sloping roof adds a ship-cabin feel.

Whether you are looking for a few finishing touches or embellishments, or are contemplating a major change in your bathroom the projects which follow should provide you with help and inspiration.

DRIFTWOOD AND SHELL FRAME

36 *B*eachcombing is an addictive pastime that can be enjoyed by all the family but, if you are regular beach visitors, the time soon comes when you need to find a use for your treasures, as all your shelves and windowsills are laden with booty. An attractive solution is to make a collage of driftwood, rope and shells into a richly textured frame for a picture or mirror. To prevent it from also being richly "fragrant", it is important to soak all the materials you use in a bleach solution for three days or so. Stand them to dry in a warm room and, if anything is still smelly, discard it. This bleaching also gives the material an attractive, sun-kissed look which is perfect for a muted-coloured bathroom.

--- ◦◎ MATERIALS ◎◦ ---
unpainted picture frame, approximately
45 × 38cm/18 × 15in, made from flat timber
about 7.5cm/3in wide
2 picture hooks
picture wire
sepia acrylic artist's ink
paint-mixing container
paintbrush
selection of shells, driftwood and rope, cleaned
(see above)
tacks
tack hammer
glue gun and hot wax glue

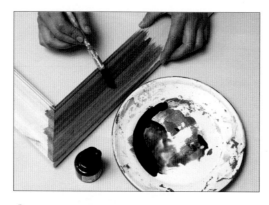

1 Attach the hooks to the back of the frame and then securely fix the wire. (This is much more difficult to do once the frame has been decorated.) Dilute the sepia ink half and half with water and brush it on to the frame. Allow to dry.

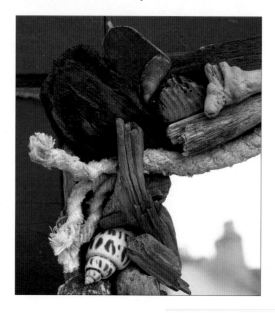

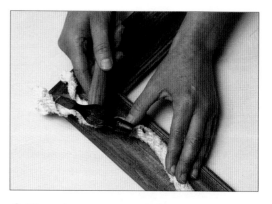

2 Place the rope around the picture frame and then tack into place.

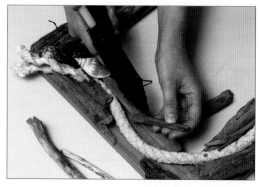

3 Work your way around the frame, firstly tacking and gluing the driftwood in place and then filling in with shells.

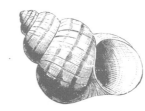

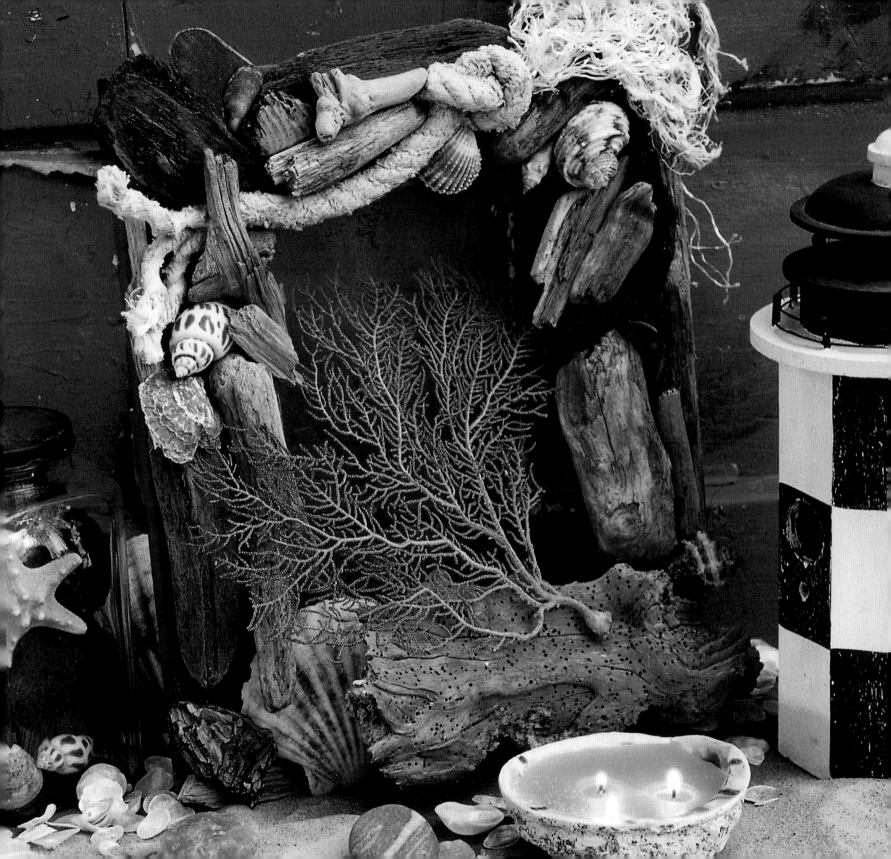

Drawstring Linen Laundry Bag

*L*aundry baskets have replaced laundry bags in many bathrooms but these are so beautiful that you may be tempted back, especially if you have a small bathroom where floor space is at a premium. Use natural fibres, such as cotton or linen or, alternatively, old thick-weave cotton towels, which can still be bought inexpensively at antique shops that specialise in fabrics. For a really classy flourish, decorate each one with the embroidered monogram of the owner.

MATERIALS

2 rectangles natural linen, 56 × 70cm/22 × 28in
2 rectangles white cotton, 56 × 70cm/22 × 28in
matching thread
3m/3½ yd soft white cord

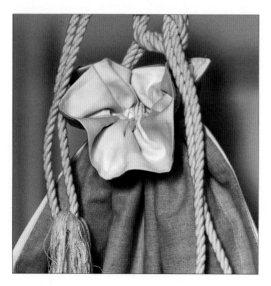

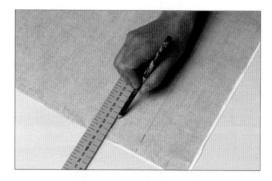

1 Place each piece of linen and of cotton together, right-sides facing. To mark the channel for the drawstrings, use a ruler to draw a pencil line 10cm/4in in from the top of the fabric.

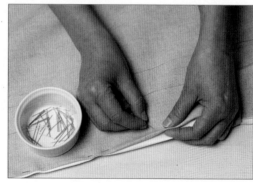

2 Draw a second line 15cm/6in from the top. Pin around the sides and the base, leaving the top open; do not pin between the pencil lines. Sew around the sides and the base, leaving the top and the marked area between the pencil lines unstitched.

3 Turn right-side out and press. Stitch along the pencil lines from one side of the rectangle to the other. This will form the channel for the cord.

Fold under the seam allowances on the raw edges, pin them together and stitch the cotton and linen together, close to the edge.

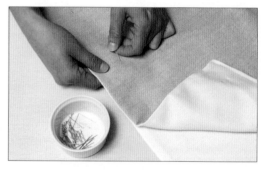

4 Press both rectangles and place one on top of the other, cotton-side inwards. Pin around the sides and the base, 5cm/2in in from the sides.

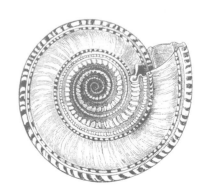

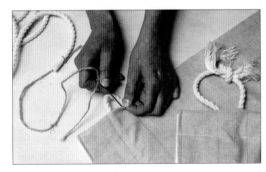

5 Stitch the sides and the base; once again, leave the cord channel unstitched. Cut the cotton cord into two equal lengths. Tie one length of cord to a piece of string or wool (yarn) threaded on to a large needle. Pull the cord through one channel, out the other side and then back through the other channel.

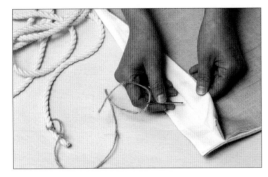

6 Tie the two ends together, using a reef knot and unravel the ends of the cord to make a tassel. Repeat this process with the other piece of cord but thread it into the channel from the other side of the bag. Pull the cords to gather the bag.

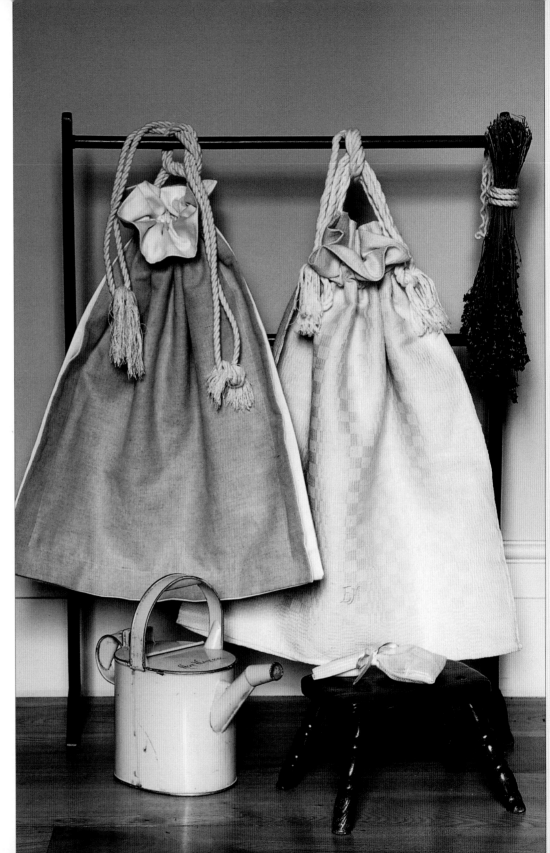

SEASHELL CANDLES

Whether you are looking for contemplative solitude or setting the scene for major seduction, a candle-lit bathroom will fulfil your requirements. The warm glow of flickering flames, reflected in tiles, taps and water, can soothe away weariness, impart a smooth, golden hue to the skin and make you feel calm and relaxed.

Candles are very easy to make, especially if shells or tiny buckets are used as moulds. When beeswax is combined with paraffin wax they will burn for a considerable length of time, allowing this to be an oft-repeated pleasure. Use a variety of shells, in different shapes and sizes, for dramatic effect. The wick used will burn a candle of up to 5cm/2in diameter, so, if the surface area is greater than this on the larger shells, add one or more extra wicks: this allows for even burning and looks very attractive.

Rather than scenting the candles with essential oils at the time of making, add a drop of oil to the pool of melted wax at the base of the wick, once the candles are lit. This allows you to change the fragrance according to your mood. Try rose geranium to lift your mood; jasmine for seduction; bergamot to calm you down. Experiment with the different oils but remember that some are much stronger than others and can be overpowering if used too liberally.

-ᴄⱻ MATERIALS ⱻᴄ-

shells in various sizes, well cleaned and dried
sand-filled bowl or plate
150g/5oz paraffin wax
50 g/2oz natural beeswax
double-boiler
metal-core wick for small candles (available from specialist suppliers)
greaseproof (waxed) paper

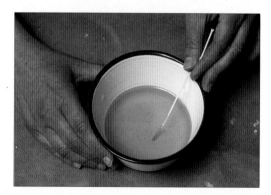

1 Place the shells in the sand-filled bowl. This will ensure that they do not tip over when filled with wax. Melt the waxes in the double-boiler and remove from the heat. Prime the wicks by soaking 15cm/6in lengths of wick in the wax for 5 minutes.

> WARNING
> Waxes *must* be melted in a double-boiler, as they are volatile and can ignite if in direct contact with heat.

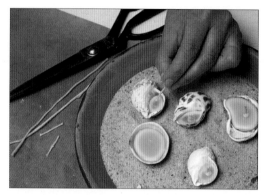

2 Allow to cool on a sheet of greaseproof (waxed) paper. If the wax has begun to set, return to the double-boiler and melt once again. Carefully pour the wax into the shells. Do not overfill or the wax will drip out of the shells when the candles are lit. Leave until the wax has partially set (small shells will set rapidly; larger ones will take proportionally longer). Push the primed wicks into the soft wax. The wick should protrude about 1cm/½ in above the wax.

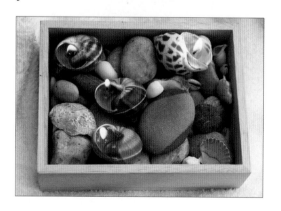

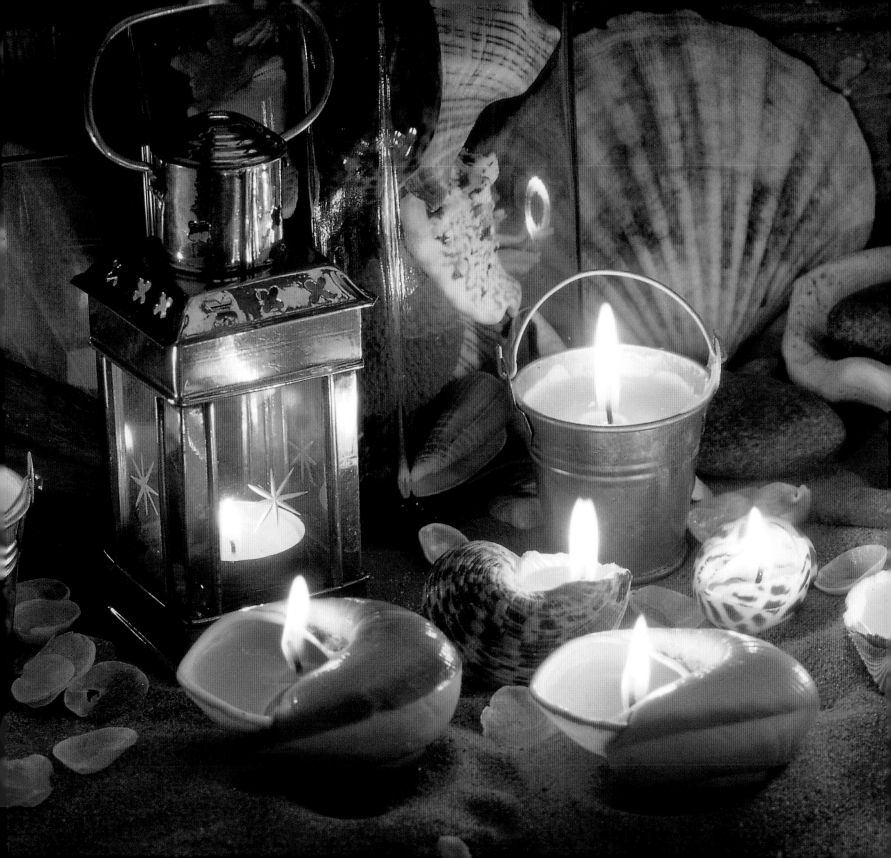

$\mathcal{A}$ water colour of an Edwardian bathing beauty provided the inspiration for the paintwork on this set of shelves.

⌐ MATERIALS ⌐
3 × 45cm/18in lengths of wood, 15cm/6in wide,
2cm/¾ in thick, for the backboards
electric drill, with 1cm/½ in routing drill bit
2 × 45cm/18in lengths of wood, 10cm/4in wide,
2cm/¾ in thick
wood glue
12 × 3cm/1½ in wood screws
candle
white and bright blue emulsion (latex) paint
paintbrush
fine-grade sandpaper
wire (steel) wool
1.5m/1¾ yd cord
scallop shell
tile cement
wax polish

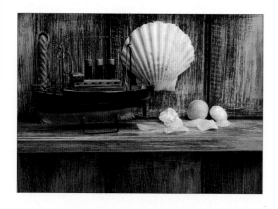

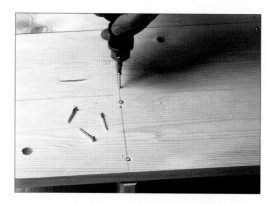

1 Referring to the template, take two of the backboards and use the routing bit to drill a hole 3cm/1½ in in from one of the corners. If you have the appropriate tools, you can round off these corners, as shown in the template, or, alternatively, you can soften the angle by rubbing the corners with sandpaper. Take the two shelves and drill a hole at each end, 2cm/¾ in in from the back and 3cm/1½ in from the side.

2 Glue the three backboards together, as shown in the template, so that the drilled holes and rounded corners are positioned in the top corners. Allow the glue to dry. Mark the position of the shelves on the backboards and glue the shelves in place. Allow the glue to dry. Carefully turn the shelves over, so that the backboards are resting on the shelves. Drill two holes through each backboard and into the shelves.

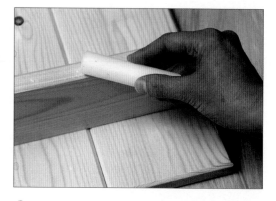

3 Screw the backboard to the shelves. Rub over the shelves with the candle, applying the wax thickly on the shelf edges and other areas where you think that wear would be most likely.

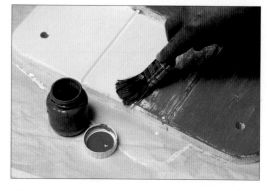

4 Paint the shelves with white emulsion (latex) paint. Allow to dry fully. Thin the blue paint to the thickness of cream, with water. Apply a coat of blue paint over the white paint and allow to dry.

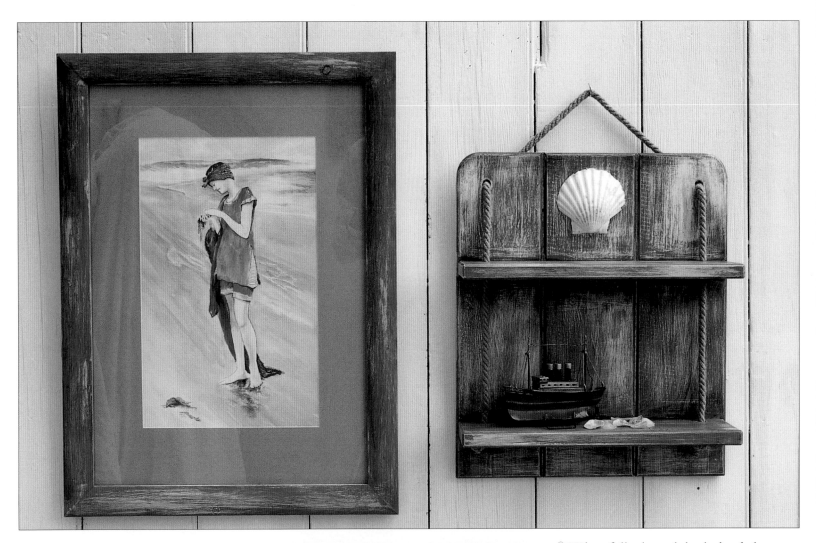

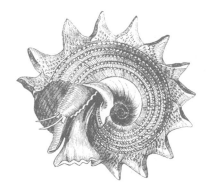

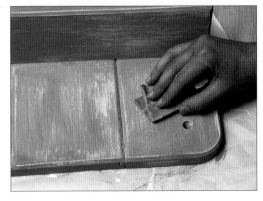

5 When fully dry, rub back the shelves with sandpaper and wire (steel) wool. Thread the cord from the back of the shelves through the holes at the top and the holes in the shelves. Knot the cord. Fill the back of the scallop shell with tile cement and leave overnight. Once it has fully hardened, smooth with sandpaper and then use more cement or glue to fasten the shell in position and apply a coat of wax polish.

A COMFORTABLE CHAIR

To contrast with the Seaside Shelves project, which showed you how to start with a new piece of furniture and age it, this project shows you how to give an old chair a new lease of life. It is a common fate of wooden chairs that have become a bit battered and out of date to be given a coat of paint and used in bathrooms or bedrooms. These often end up in junk shops, where they can be bought for next to nothing.

Before buying a chair, do try sitting in it to check that it is comfortable and that there are no sharp edges. The chair used in this project is an old bentwood chair with its original cane back and, although the cane seat has been replaced by wood, its proportions are still lovely. Some ingrained paint has been left, to give the chair the appearance of limed wood. The addition of a padded cushion on the seat makes it a comfortable and attractive bathroom chair. Whether the cushion is bought or home-made, bear in mind the damp atmosphere of a bathroom and make sure it is filled with foam or wadding (batting), rather than feathers.

WARNING
NB: Wear rubber gloves at all times
when using paint stripper

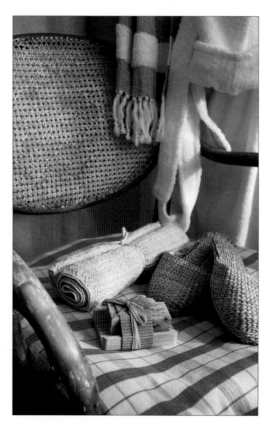

--◦ MATERIALS ◦--
painted chair
paint stripper
rubber gloves
paintbrush
stripping knife
wire pot-scourer
fine-grade sandpaper
wire (steel) wool
wax polish

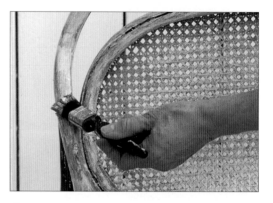

1 Place the chair on a protected surface in a well ventilated room and paint it generously with paint stripper, following the manufacturer's instructions and wearing rubber gloves. It may be necessary to apply the paint stripper two or three times, depending on how many layers of paint there are on the chair.

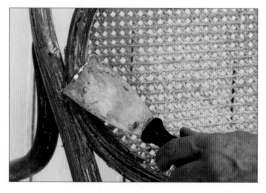

2 Use the stripping knife to remove paint from the chair. Leave some traces of paint if you wish to give an attractive finish.

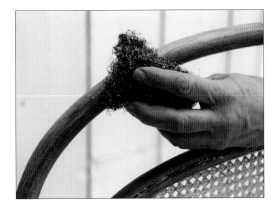

3 Use the wire pot-scourer on the areas that cannot be reached by the knife.

4 When you have removed the required amount of paint, wash the chair to remove any paint stripper. Leave to dry.

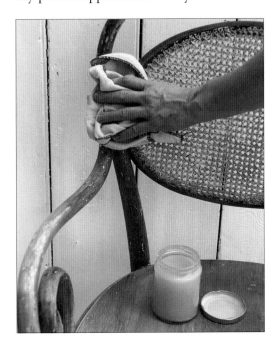

5 Gently sand the surfaces, to remove any roughness and then rub over with wire (steel) wool. Give it a coat of wax polish.

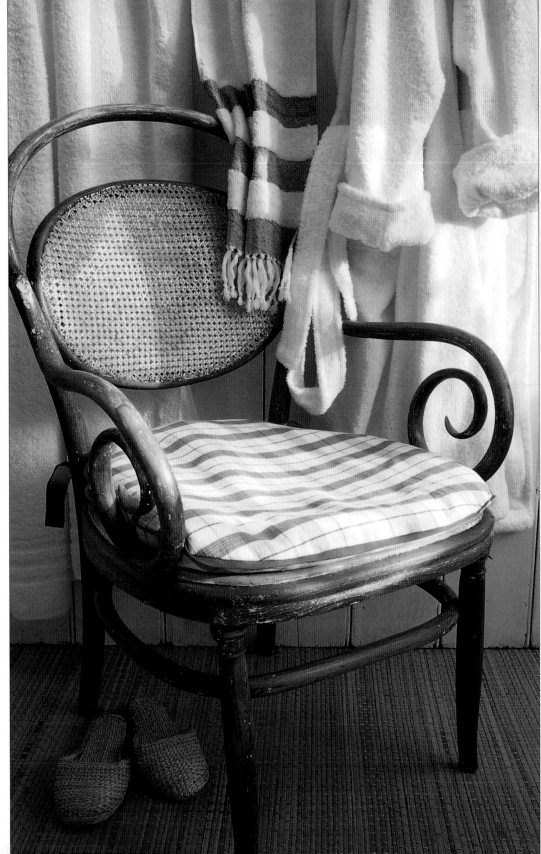

SCANDINAVIAN PAINTED FLOOR

46

This painted floor has all the appearance of wooden boards but is, in fact, made from strips of hardboard that have been painted and grained with a comb before the application of a decorative paint finish and a sealing coat of varnish. Although you may need some professional help laying the boards, you will have an attractive and durable floor at a fraction of the usual price. Practise using the comb, it is easy but needs to be used with confidence. Hold the comb firmly at one end of the board and, as you move it down the board, gently and slowly rock it on its curved surface and you will see the graining pattern appear. Vary the design by running the comb once down some of the boards and twice down others. As the comb is used on wet paint, the board can be repainted if you aren't happy with the results.

This type of floor is ideal when an existing wooden floor is in poor condition. Single overlapping sheets of newspaper can be placed over the existing floor, to even out any lumps and bumps. The boards could also be laid on a solid surface, using a suitable adhesive. Provided that the floor is sealed with flexible sealant between the boards and finished with a couple of coats of varnish, it will be waterproof and reasonably hard wearing. Renew the varnish after a couple of years.

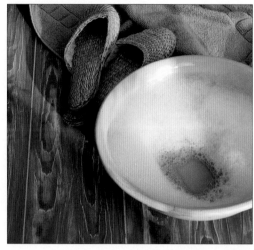

MATERIALS

good-quality, off-white matt emulsion paint
paintbrushes
6mm/½ in hardboard sheets, cut into 15cm/6in
wide boards
wood graining comb
jade green matt emulsion paint
paint-mixing container
fine-grade sandpaper
cloth
quick-drying satin varnish
saw
2cm/¾ in oblong nails
hammer
nail-punch
flexible acrylic sealant
sponge

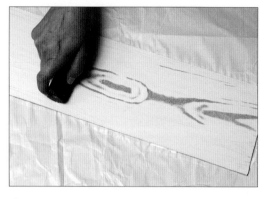

1 Paint a thick coat of the off-white emulsion on to the boards and, while the paint is still wet, run the graining comb down the length of each board to create the "grain". Allow to dry.

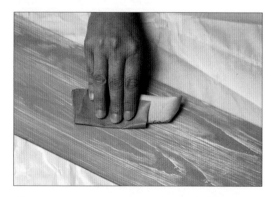

2 Mix the jade paint with water to the consistency of cream and paint a thin coat on the "grained" boards. Allow to dry. Rub over the boards with sandpaper to remove the wash from the "grain" underneath and reveal some of the lighter-coloured paint.

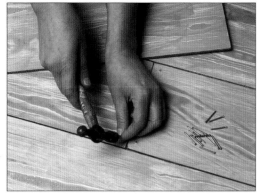

3 Wipe the boards with a damp cloth and seal with a coat of varnish. Allow to dry. Cut the boards to size and lay out on the floor, leaving a small gap between the boards. Lay the floor using oblong nails.

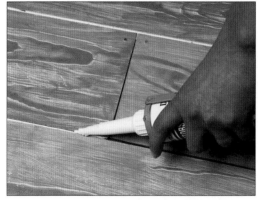

4 Use a punch to ensure that the nail heads are below the floor surface. Seal the gap between the boards with acrylic sealant. Use a damp sponge to smooth the sealant and wipe away any excess. Leave to dry. Finally paint on two more coats of varnish, allowing the floor to dry thoroughly between coats.

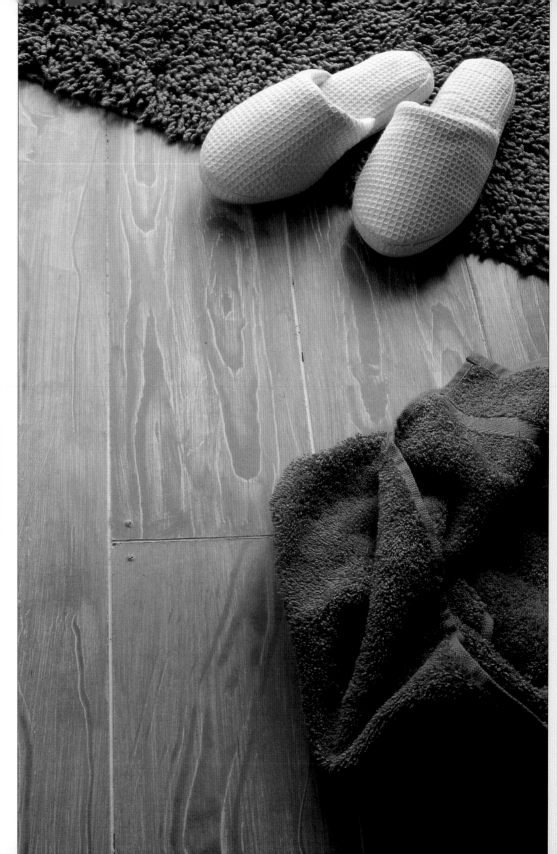

SEAWEED AND SHELL COLLAGE PICTURES

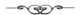

48

Seaweed and shell pictures were very popular in Victorian times, when ladies would spend many hours assembling ornate and intricate collages that would then be framed with uplifting or sentimental verses. Nowadays, we have neither the time nor the inclination for such pastimes but these simplified versions of those earlier pictures are both quick and easy to make and extremely stylish. In one of the pictures, the seaweed is held in place by an attractively marked shell, while the other uses a tiny woven basket to contain the seaweed. Both are labelled with the place and date they were collected and they would be lovely mementoes of a visit to the beach.

—◦ MATERIALS ◦—

seaweed
cream card (cardboard), cut to fit
glue gun and hot wax glue
scissors
small woven basket or shell
label
display frame

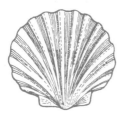

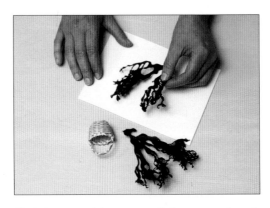

1 Select suitable pieces of the seaweed and move them around on the card (cardboard) until you have formed a fan-shaped spray you are happy with. Glue in position.

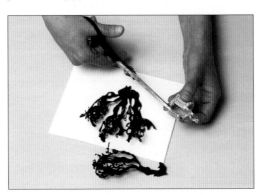

2 Use scissors to cut the back third off the basket and then fold under the raw edges. If using a shell, it should be a cockle or similar shape, which is flat enough to glue securely to the card.

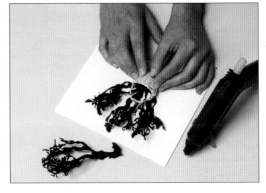

3 Glue the basket in position over the spray of seaweed. Hold it in position until the glue has dried.

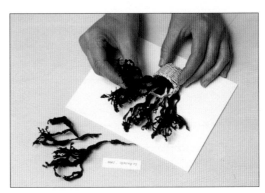

4 Tuck more sprays of seaweed into the front of the basket.

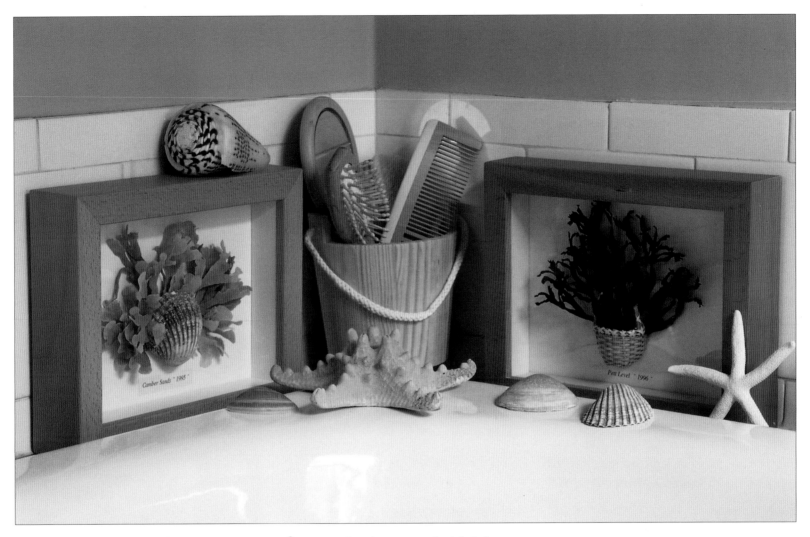

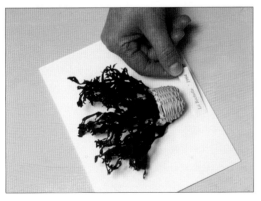

5 Type or hand-write on the label the details of where the seaweed was collected. Add the label to the collage and place the picture in the display frame.

RIGHT: Plastic fish brought from a toy shop swim menacingly underneath a fishing boat on a painted background in this picture frame. Create your own designs, adding 1 and 2 dimensional features for interesting effect.

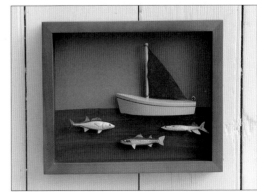

STARFISH TILES

Stamping is an extremely easy way to add colour and design to plain tiles. The range of stamps available is huge and there are many, like this starfish, which are ideal for bathrooms. The plain border on the tile is applied with the roller, following pencil guidelines, while the more time-consuming checkerboard design has been hand-painted over a pencilled pattern. Ceramic paint is used to stamp the design on the tile and, once the design is dry, it can be cleaned (but not with an abrasive cleaning product). If you would like the design to be more durable, bake the tiles in the oven, following the paint-manufacturer's instructions.

Adding a stamped border or design is also an ideal way to change the look of an existing bathroom. Plan your design first, by marking the chosen tiles with a chinagraph

pencil and, once you are happy with the balance of patterned and plain tiles, start stamping. Don't worry about variation of colour tone caused by the amount of paint loaded on the roller: this gives the tiles a hand-made look, which usually costs a lot more than mass-manufactured tiles! Any disasters can be put right with white spirit (turpentine), provided that the paint has not dried.

-- MATERIALS --
chinagraph pencil
ruler
white ceramic tiles
starfish stamp
roller
green ceramic paint
tin plate
white spirit

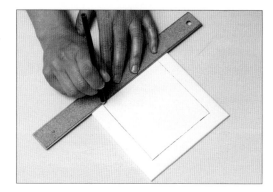

1 Draw the pencil guidelines for the border on the tiles.

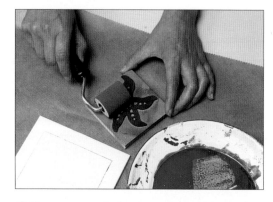

2 Pour some of the ceramic paint into the tin plate and load the roller, by pushing it backwards and forwards. When it is evenly coated, roll the paint on to the stamp.

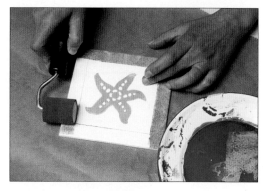

3 Push the stamp firmly on to the surface of the tile, being careful that it does not slip. Lift the stamp away from the tile. Leave to dry. Following the guidelines, use the roller to paint the border around the tile. When you have finished clean the stamp and roller with white spirit (turpentine).

50

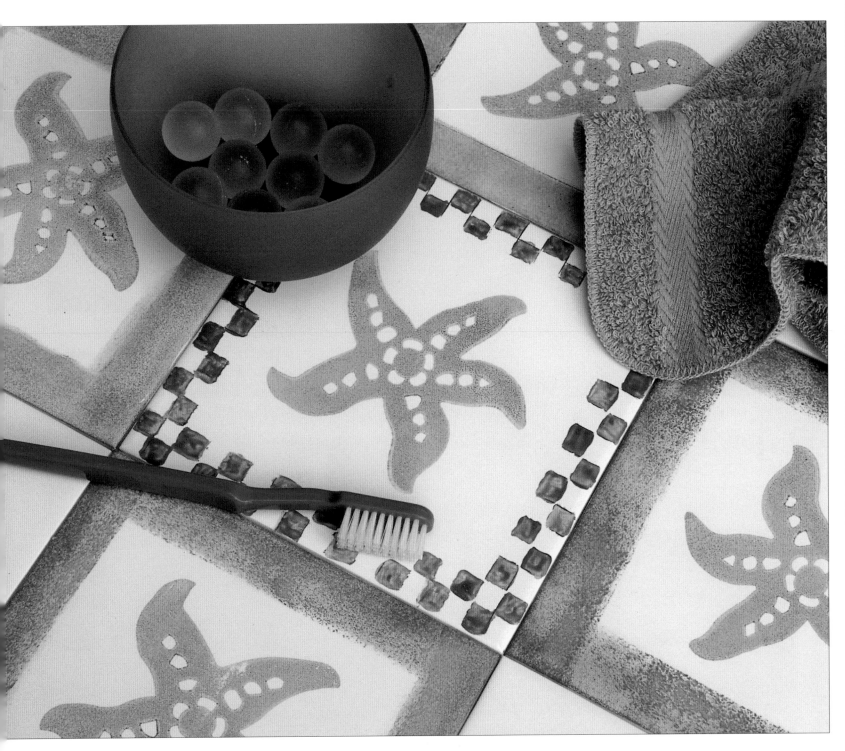

COUNTRY-STYLE CUPBOARD

52 Bathroom cupboards need to be practical and functional, a place to put all those bits and pieces that seem to gather in quantity in the bathroom; but there is no reason why they cannot be pretty as well. The inside of this cupboard has been lined with a pretty wrapping paper, featuring small designs, including the fish, some of which were cut out to decorate the exterior of the cupboard. Wallpaper could be used instead but be sure to choose a paper that is to scale with the cupboard for the best effect.

MATERIALS

small pine cupboard
fine-grade sandpaper
cream and pale green emulsion (latex) paint
paintbrushes
wrapping paper or wallpaper
tape measure
scissors
wallpaper paste
wax crayon
matt varnish

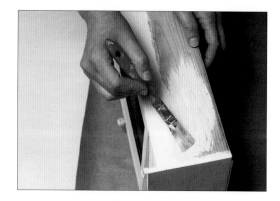

1 Rub the surface of the cupboard with sandpaper, to remove any polish or dirt before painting. Wipe off any dust with a dry cloth. Paint the exterior of the cupboard lightly with cream paint. Allow to dry. Rub down with sandpaper, so that the grain of the wood is revealed in places.

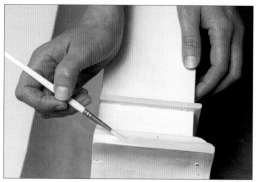

2 Pick out the moulding and the door frame in green. Allow to dry and sand again, until you have achieved a slightly distressed look that you like.

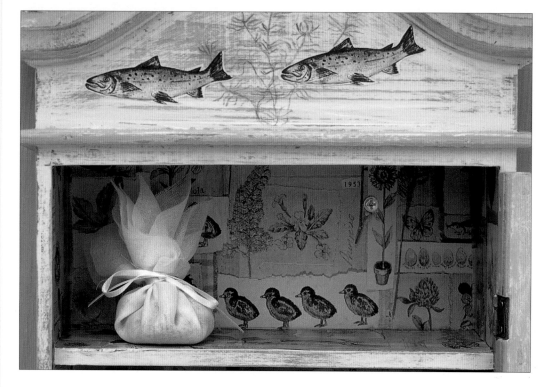

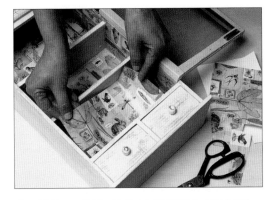

3 Cut the wrapping or wallpaper to fit the shelves and attach it to the cupboard, using wallpaper paste.

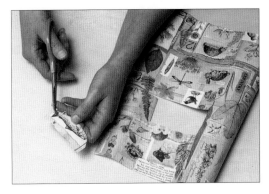

4 Choose a motif from the paper, in this instance the fish, cut it out carefully and use to decorate the exterior of the cupboard. The pondweed behind the fish has been drawn in using a crayon. The cupboard has then been painted inside and out with two coats of matt varnish, to seal and protect the paper and the paint.

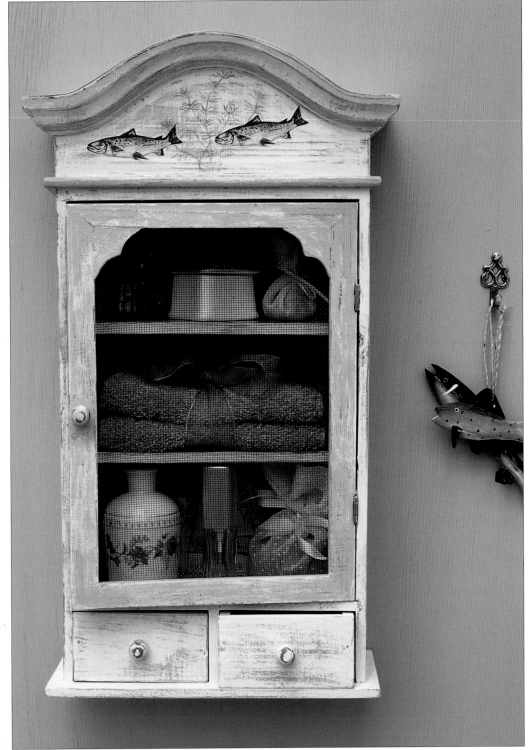

PRETTILY PAINTED GLASS

Special glass paints in vibrant colours are now readily available and with them you can transform an ordinary bottle into something fit for a genie. There are two types of paint, thin translucent paint for fine detail and stained-glass colours and a thicker-textured opaque paint in gold, silver or black, which can be used to outline or create a relief design. This project describes the method for a checkerboard-design glass jar but with these two types of paint you can use your imagination to come up with endless ways to transform glass jars and bottles.

Experiment on an old jam jar before you begin, to get the feel of the materials. Once you have started correct any mistakes using a cotton-wool bud dipped in white spirit (turpentine). Jars like the ones used in this project can be bought very cheaply and transformed into wonderful presents using glass paints.

‑◦ *MATERIALS* ◦‑
gold outliner
glass jar, well washed and dried
paper towel
fine paintbrush
turquoise glass paint
white spirit (turpentine)

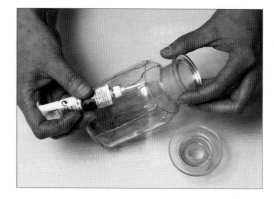

1 Use the gold outliner directly from the tube, to draw the checkerboard pattern on the jar. Have a paper towel at hand, to wipe the nozzle of the tube if there is a build-up of paint around it. Allow to dry fully, overnight if possible.

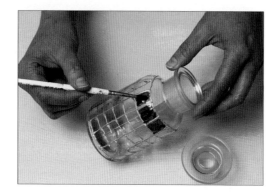

2 Using the fine paintbrush, fill in the squares with the turquoise glass paint. For more intense colour, apply a second coat of paint once the first has dried. Wash the brush in white spirit (turpentine).

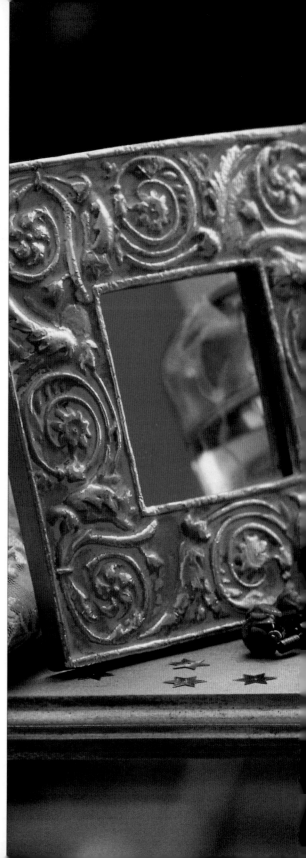

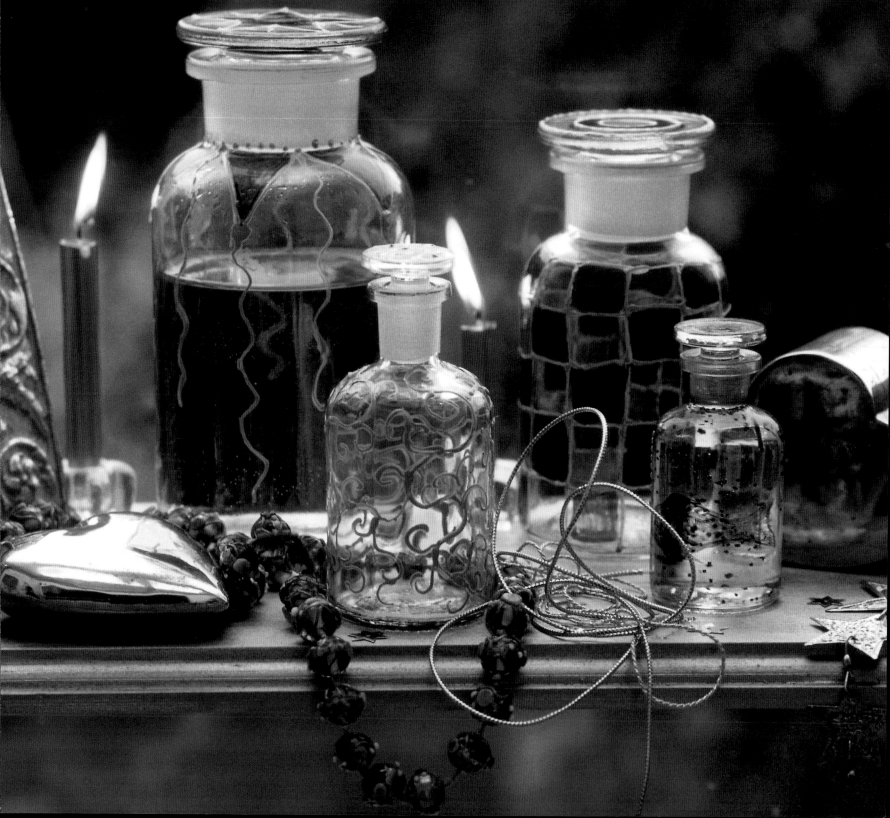

JAUNTY TOWELS

*I*nspired by the flotilla of jolly sailing boats above the row of hooks and further complementing the marine theme in this bathroom, boats have been appliquéd on to royal-blue hand towels and turquoise bath towels. The simple outlines have been cut from cotton piqué and sewn on to the towels, using a zigzag stitch. It is a good idea to use thread the same colour as the towel in the bobbin of the machine, so that the stitching does not stand out on the reverse side of the towels but you can use a contrasting thread if you prefer.

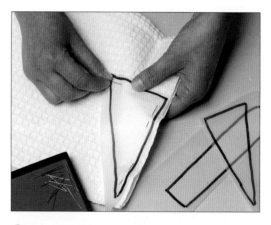

2 Cut out the paper-pattern pieces and pin them on to the cotton piqué fabric.

→∘ MATERIALS ∘←

tracing paper
pencil
scissors
dressmaker's pins
0.5m / ½ yd white cotton piqué
0.5m / ½ yd royal-blue cotton piqué
2 royal-blue cotton hand towels
2 turquoise-blue bath towels
sewing machine
matching or contrasting thread

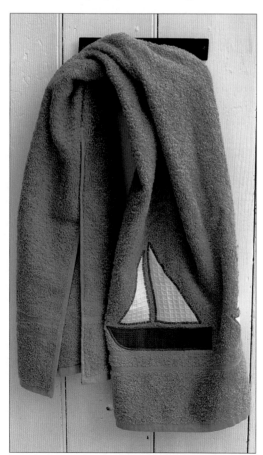

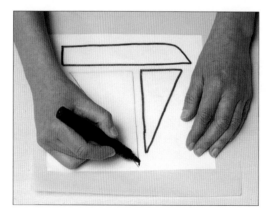

1 Use tracing paper and pencil to trace the template of the sailing boat.

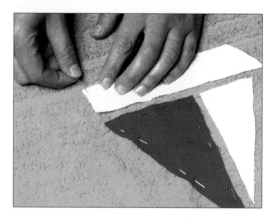

3 Cut out the fabric pieces, remove the tracing paper and pin the fabric pieces to the towel. Stitch round the pattern pieces, using a dense zigzag stitch, in matching or contrasting thread, as you prefer.

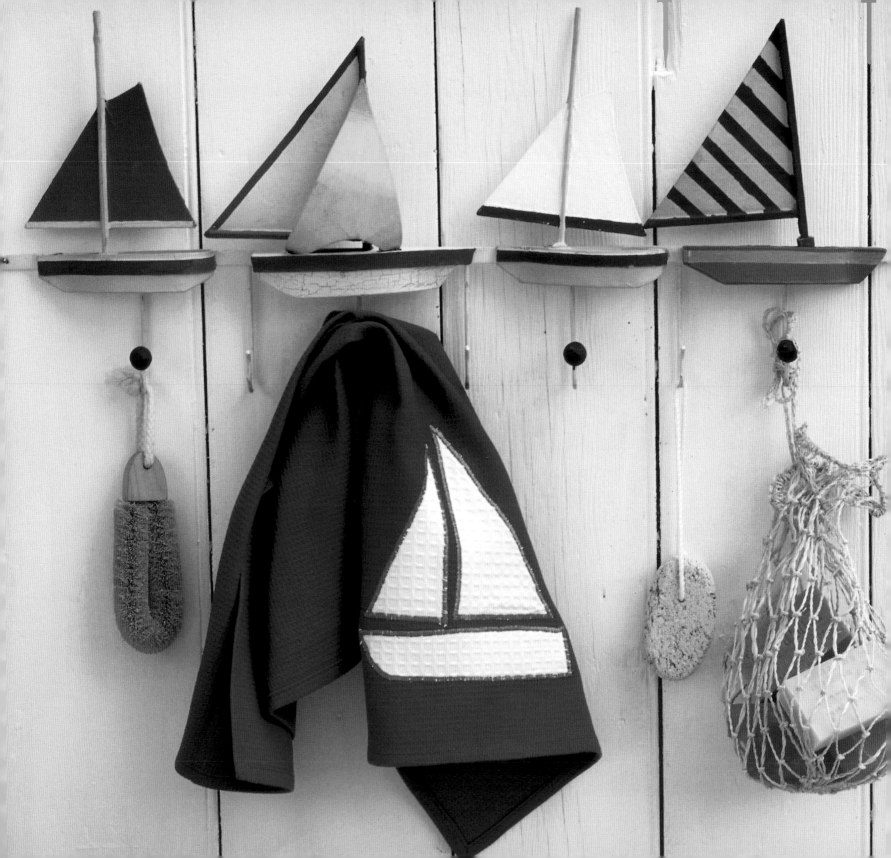

WIRE BATH TIDY

58

*T*his wire tidy is ideal for storing all the brushes, sponges and loofahs that need to dry out thoroughly between use. Inspired by the inventive use craft workers make of everyday materials, this tidy is made in minutes from galvanised wire netting and raffia. Care has been taken to ensure that there are no sharp edges but, even so, this is not recommended for the bathrooms of families with small children. Filled with a variety of natural sponges and a selection of wood-backed brushes, the tidy would make a lovely gift for a friend's bathroom.

∼◦ MATERIALS ◦∼
small-gauge galvanised chicken wire
wire cutters or secateurs
natural raffia
large-eyed needle

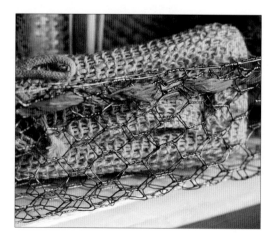

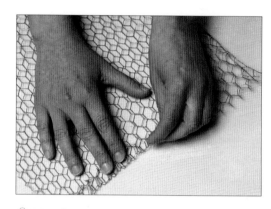

1 Use the wire cutters or secateurs to cut a 50cm/20in length of chicken wire. Fold it in half lengthways, so that the smooth edges meet. Fold over the cut ends at either end, to make them smooth as well.

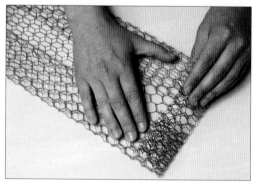

2 Fold the wire over on itself, on all four sides. The folds should be 7.5cm/3in deep.

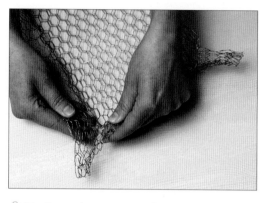

3 To form the corners of the tidy first press the folds firmly to ensure sharp creases and then unfold and open out the corners. Fold the opened-out corners flat against the long sides of the tidy.

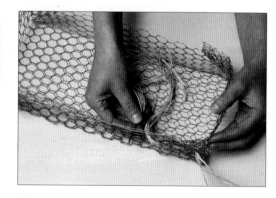

4 Thread two or three lengths of raffia on to the needle and use to make running stitches round the edge of the tidy, from corner to corner. Where the raffia meets at the corners, tie a reef knot and trim the ends.

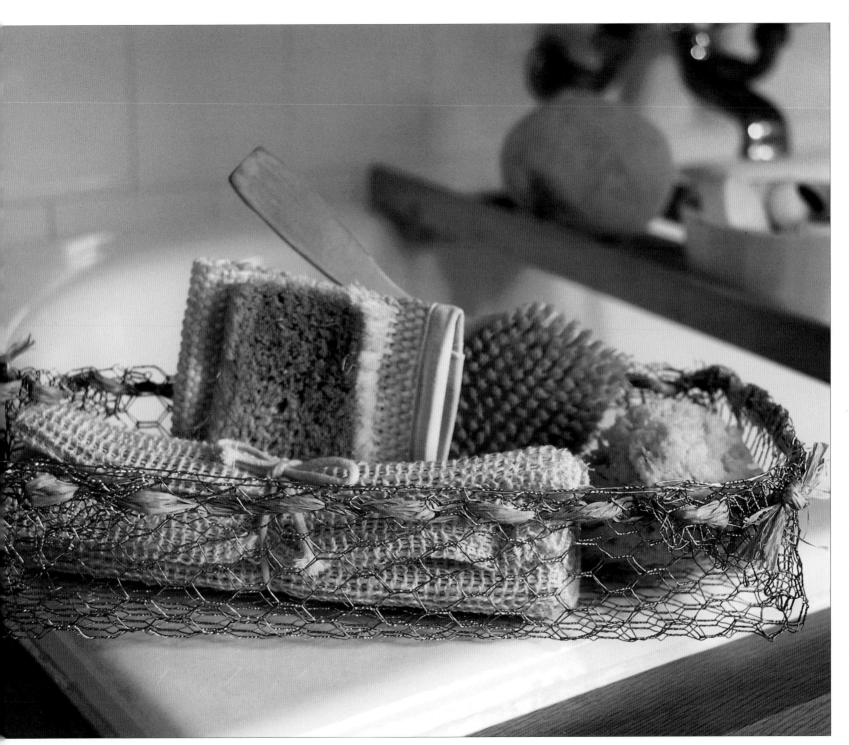

NEO-CLASSICAL BLIND

Bold designs can be painted on to a plain blind, to add drama to the bathroom. The inspiration for this neo-classical urn is to be found on the patterned voile curtains that surround the window. A simplified version of one of the designs on the fabric has been traced on to paper and then enlarged, using a photocopier. If you do not have access to a photocopier, high-street stationery or print shops will do this for you. The urn has then been traced on to the blind and painted using fabric paints. Fabric paints usually come in fairly strong colours and, to achieve more subtle colouring, are mixed with a "medium," which softens the colour without thinning the paint. Check in craft shops for the paints and medium. If the urn design does not appeal to you, look at fabrics, pictures or wallpapers for your inspiration and take a tracing of the design you like.

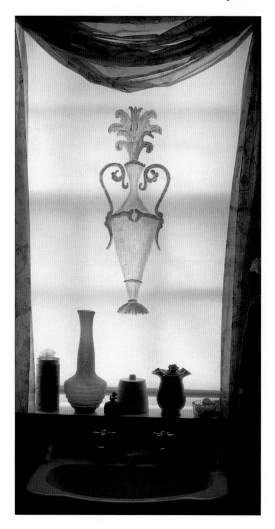

MATERIALS

tracing paper
pencil
soft pencil
fabric paints and medium
paint-mixing container
paintbrushes
iron

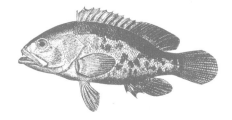

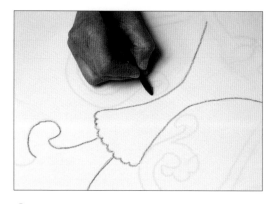

1 Trace the pattern from the template at the back of the book. Enlarge the design to the required size, using a photocopier. Trace the design directly on to the blind, using a soft pencil.

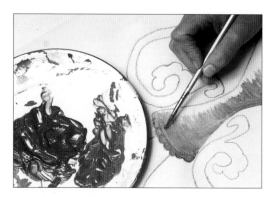

2 Mix the paints to the required shades, with the medium, and paint the design on to the blind. When the paint is dry, press the reverse side of the blind with a hot iron, to fix the design and remove any wrinkles.

SCALLOP SHELL BIN

*A*traditional, galvanized bucket has been given a classical découpage decoration of scallop shells, to transform it from the mundane to the refined. Use it to store towels or as an attractive but practical waste bin. The shell design is photocopied from the template and then carefully cut out, before being mounted on the bucket and sealed with varnish. As varnish tends to yellow slightly with age, it is best to varnish the whole of the bucket exterior.

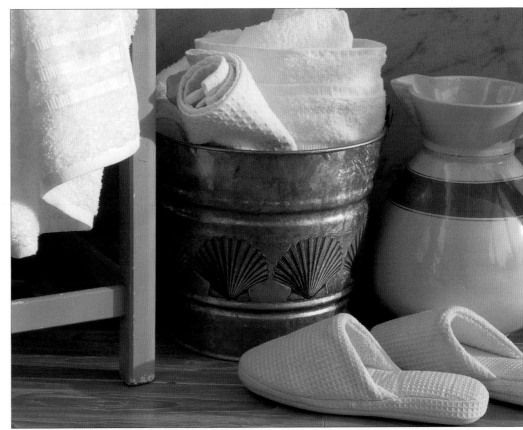

❧ MATERIALS ❧
sharp scissors
wallpaper paste
galvanised bucket
dry cloth
paintbrush
quick-drying clear matt varnish

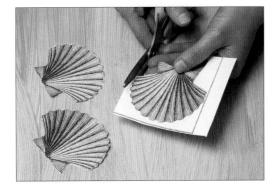

1 Carefully cut out 8 scallop shells using photocopies of the templates at the back of the book.

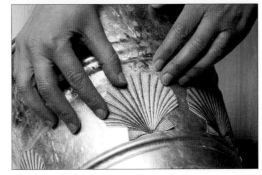

2 Paint the reverse of the shells with wallpaper paste and position them on the bucket. Gently but firmly press the shells with a dry cloth, to remove any air bubbles. Leave to dry. Give the bucket at least three coats of varnish, to seal and protect the scallop shells.

MERMAID SHOWER CURTAIN

Muslin may seem to be the most impractical of fabrics for a shower curtain but, when backed with an opaque waterproof liner, you can make shower curtains from any fabric. For this project, natural muslin has been decorated with gilded mermaids and dyed a soft sea green, to create an unusual and softly sumptuous shower curtain. To keep the mermaids' bodies free of colour, the fabric has been painted with a resist medium to ensure that the dye does not take on these areas. Cold-water dye has been used and the fabric was hand-dyed to give the random "watery" effect.

8m/8yd muslin
black permanent marker pen
resist medium
iron
sea-green cold-water dye
dye fixative
cloth
gold contour-lining fabric paint
shower-curtain liner
sewing machine
dressmaker's pins
matching thread
2m/2yd net curtain header tape
2m/2yd self-adhesive Velcro tape

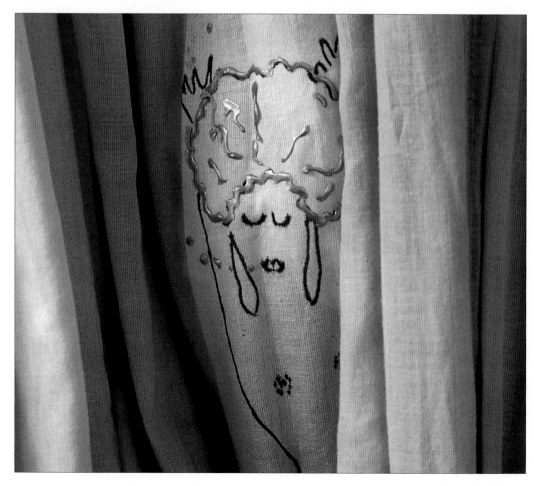

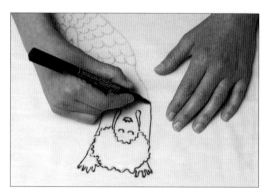

1 Cut the muslin into four 2m/2yd lengths and mark the position of the mermaids. Photocopy the mermaid template. Lay each piece of muslin over the photocopy and use the marker pen to draw the outline of the mermaids.

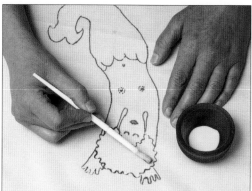

2 Paint the whole area of the upper body of each mermaid with resist medium and allow to dry. Press through a cloth with a hot iron for 2 minutes, to fix. Loosely fold the fabric and hand-dye it according to the dye-manufacturer's instructions, using the fixative at the end of the process. Iron the fabric when dry.

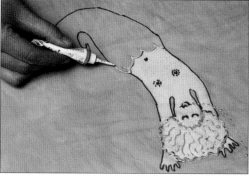

3 Paint in the hair and scales of the mermaid, with the gold contour paint, and add bubbles. Allow to dry flat. Pin together and make up the muslin panels to the same size as the liner. Gather the fabric tightly on to net curtain header tape. Attach the curtain and the liner with the Velcro strip.

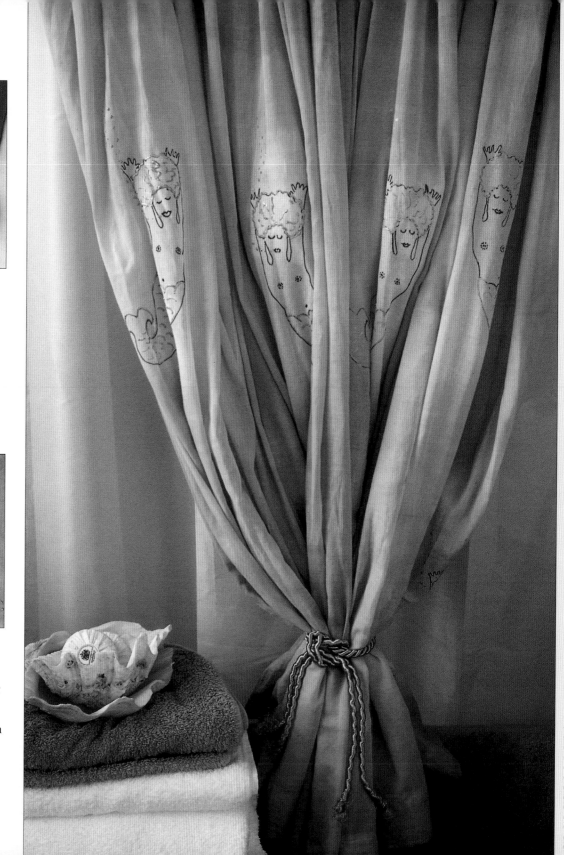

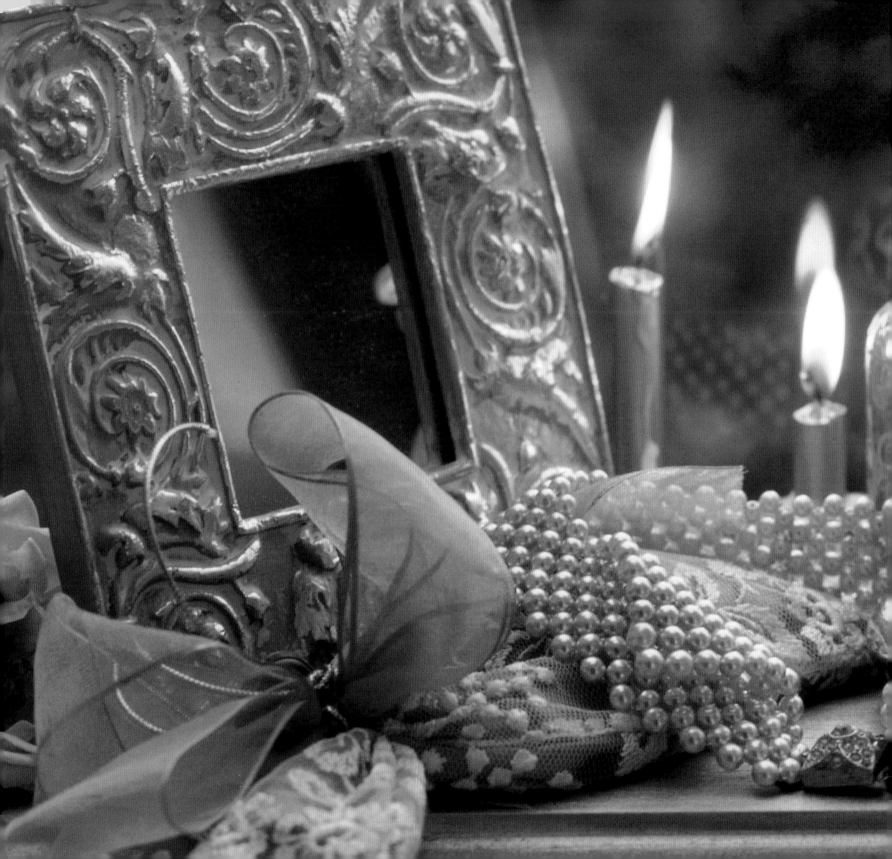

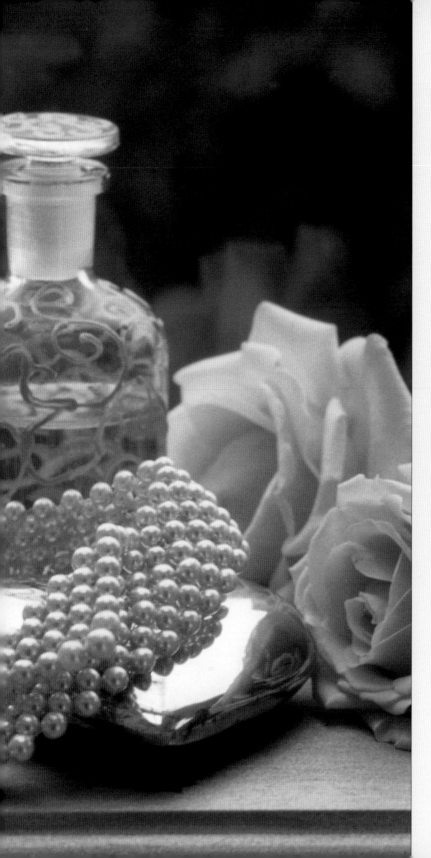

Chapter Three

BATHING

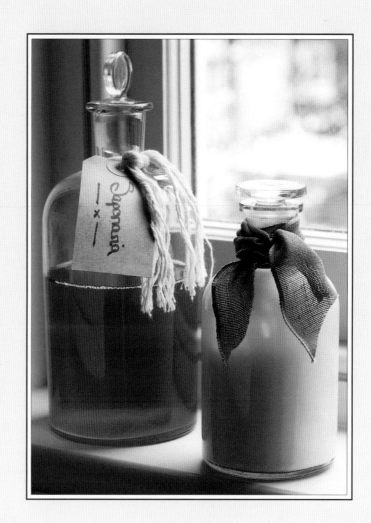

ABOVE: *Pure natural ingredients are all that are needed to make a wide range*

of bath products and cosmetics.

LEFT: *Soft candlelight is reflected in the mirror and bottles.*

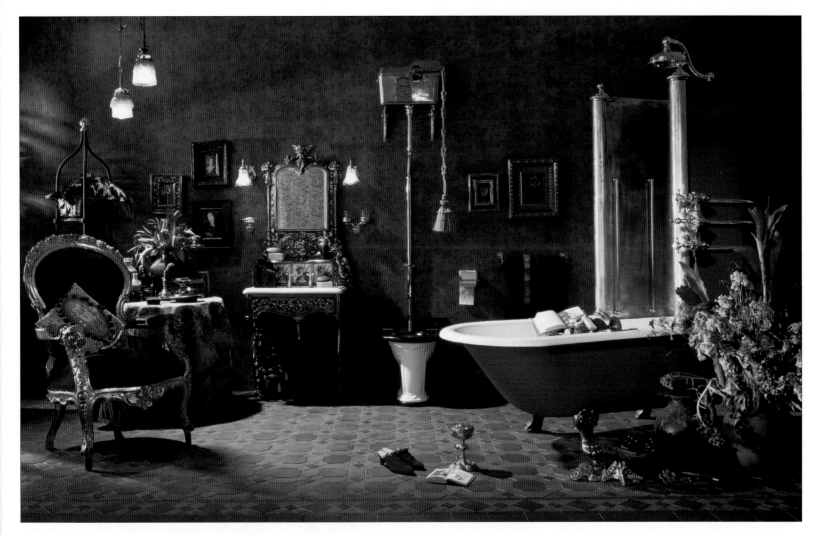

*B*athing is about so much more than cleanliness. It is as much a ritual as a routine – the bathroom becomes a sanctuary where pampering is permitted and privacy is generally respected.

In our busy lives, many of us choose to shower, well aware that the seductive pleasures of the bath will slow us down and dilute our sense of urgency, for when we immerse ourselves in water we return to the element in which we began our life and we are soothed and comforted. But, even in the busiest life, there are still moments when only a bath will do. In the absence of time to take a holiday, visit a health spa or take a day off, we can retreat behind the bathroom door, run a deep, scented bath and sink beneath the water to emerge later, rested and relaxed and with renewed energy for life's hustle and bustle.

We all have our own vision of our dream

ABOVE: With a bathroom like this, one could revive the custom of bathing in the company of friends.

bathroom and some of us may realize that dream; all of us, however, can transform the bathroom we already own into a personal oasis, where we can learn to enjoy the rituals of the bath. The transformation requires inspiration rather than time or money and will add immeasurably to your pleasure. Just

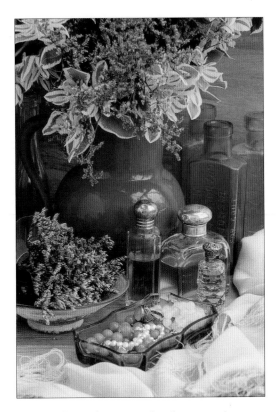

ABOVE: Flowers bring a touch of luxury to the bathroom as do decorative glass and china.

as a successful night out can benefit from a bit of forward planning, so a night in can be something special with a little forethought.

~ WARMTH ~

However beautiful your bathroom may be, it is difficult to enjoy the full sybaritic pleasure of bathing if the air or water temperature is not sufficiently warm for your comfort.

An hour before you plan to bathe, check the bathroom and, if necessary, turn up the water temperature and the heating and inform the rest of the household of your plans, to ensure that they don't nip in before you and colonize your sanctuary. Drape your biggest, fluffiest towels and a bathrobe over a heated towel rail or radiator to ensure that stepping from the bath is a pleasure, not a penance (if you don't own big, fluffy towels, buy some or ask for some as a present: they are essential equipment for an indulgent bath). Similarly, towelling bathrobes should be enormous: ignore your usual sizing and buy the largest size available; a bathrobe should reach the floor and have generous folds to trap the warmth radiating from your body.

~ LIGHT ~

All who have swum by moonlight know the magical transformation that takes place when soft light and water meet. We feel the sensuous caress of the water more intensely than we ever do in daylight and our other senses are similarly enhanced. Few of us regret the advent of electric light, but not enough of us experience the pleasures of candlelight and its ability to transform an everyday experience into something special. The most ordinary of bathrooms can become an enchanted place when lit by candles whose light softly reflects in taps and tiles and twinkles on the surface of the water. Obviously, one must be very aware that combining candles and bare flesh requires a degree of caution – floating candles in the bath is not recommended – but the hand basin could contain a flotilla of floating lights, and ledges and shelves can accommodate

BELOW: Whether bathing alone or in company it is always better by candlelight.

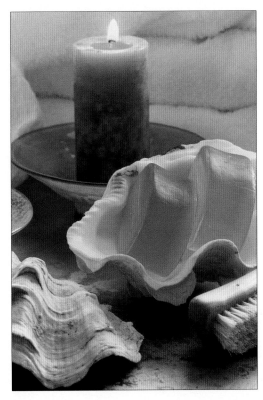

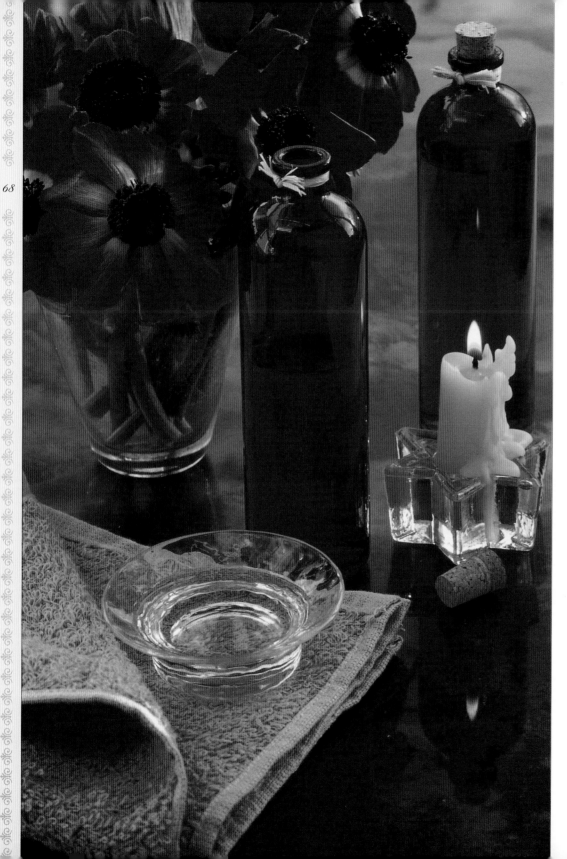

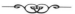

candles. Wall sconces are particularly successful in bathrooms. If candles really do
make you nervous, contain them in an assort-
ment of decorative lanterns. These are
increasingly popular and can be bought with
plain, engraved or coloured glass.

❧ SCENT ❧

Most underrated of all the senses, our sense
of smell is central to all pleasure. It is the only
one of the senses that goes straight to the
emotions without first being interpreted by
the intellect. This is why fragrance is so evoca-
tive and explains why past happiness or
unhappiness can be instantly conjured up by
a scent. Love it or hate it, your reaction to a
smell is always emotional, and choosing the
right fragrance is an important step in setting
the mood when you have pampering in mind.

Try to ensure that any fragrances you use
harmonize: the bath oil, soap, shampoo, talcum powder, deodorant, body lotion and
many other lotions and potions used in the
bathroom may each feature a different fragrance and the resultant blend is not always
successful. One of the great advantages of
adding your own essential oils to unscented
or home-made beauty products is that you

*LEFT: Scented oils can be used for massage and for
adding to the bath.*

can control the blend of fragrances or even choose a single scent, such as rose or jasmine. For a truly hedonistic experience, scent the candles with a few drops of your chosen fragrance and have a vase of roses or a jasmine plant in the bathroom.

➤ MUSIC ➤

As the fragrance of the scented water wafts upward and the gentle candlelight casts a golden glow, what better time to listen to a favourite piece of music or a reading from some sublime poetry or prose? Add an extra dimension to the atmosphere by playing tapes of ambient sounds from the rainforest or the seashore. The most sophisticated bathrooms have speakers built into the walls, but if this is beyond your means you can still enjoy the experience with the help of a battery-powered tape recorder. As most bathrooms are fairly small and have plenty of tiled surfaces, their acoustics are generally good enough to produce an enjoyable sound.

➤ TASTE ➤

This pampering of the senses should not exclude taste, and you must remember not to neglect the palate: picture yourself lifting a

RIGHT: Scented flowers are wonderful in the bathroom, fill a vase with them and float a few petals in the bath.

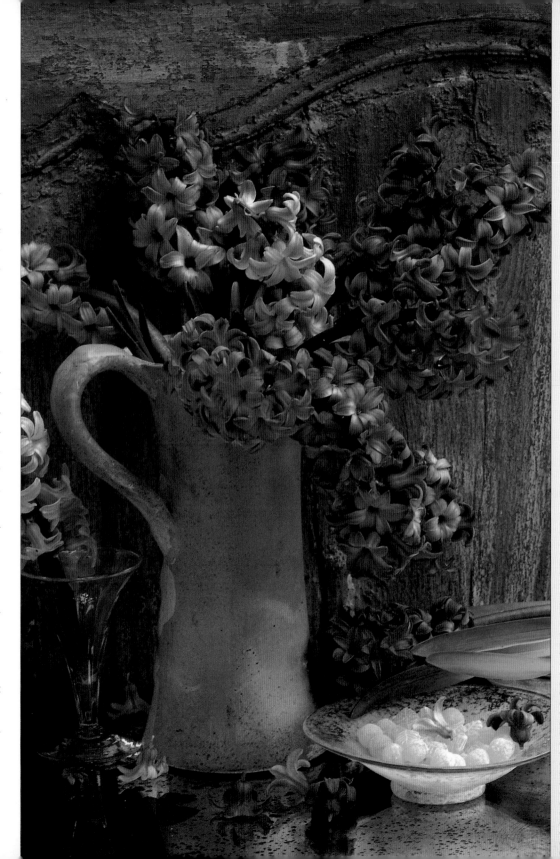

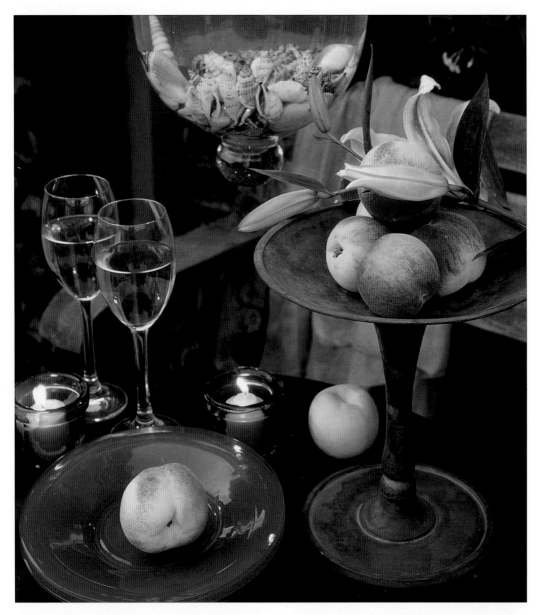

ABOVE: After a stressful day, unwind in the bath with a glass of wine and some luscious fruit.

languorous arm to reach for a chilled glass of white wine or a plump peach to complete the picture of delicious self-indulgence. There is a tendency to feel guilty about self-indulgence but setting aside time for oneself is vital to health and well-being and there is no reason why that time should be Spartan or tedious.

TOUCH

The sensation of warm water against the skin; of fluffy towels enveloping the body; of scented lotions smoothed on soft skin: all these and more are a vital part of enjoyable bathing. The Egyptians, Greeks and Romans understood and appreciated the therapeutic and sensual pleasures of the rituals of the bath and, although we certainly do not have the slaves and may not even have a willing companion to minister to our every need or capricious whim, we can take time to enjoy pampering ourselves. There is a world of difference between hurriedly applying a cream or lotion or quickly moisturizing your face, and the alternative of gently massaging it into the skin. The skin is the largest organ of the body and every bit of it is capable of feeling sensation and benefiting from touch.

In this chapter, you will find projects that use wholesome natural ingredients and fragrant essential oils to make a variety of cleansing and moisturising creams, lotions and soaps, as well as colognes and scented oils which will help enhance your enjoyment of the rituals of bathing. Fill your bathroom with these products and you will be ready to pamper yourself from top to toe, and feel the benefits afterwards as your body and mind are soothed and relaxed.

The Safe Use of Natural Products

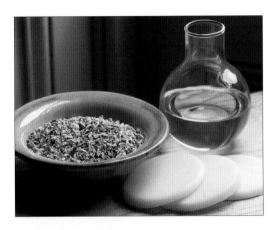

ABOVE: Soapwort root, almond oil and white beeswax are all used in natural cosmetics.

∞ HOW TO CARRY OUT A SIMPLE ∞ PATCH TEST

Take a small amount of the substance you wish to test and spread it on the sensitive skin of the inner arm. Leave it overnight and, next day, check for any sign of irritation.

∞ SAFE USE OF ESSENTIAL OILS ∞

Store essential oils out of the reach of children, in a cool, dark cupboard. Oils should not be used undiluted – the only exception is lavender oil, which can be used on minor cuts or burns. They must be mixed with a "base" or "carrier" oil before being applied to the skin, or they will cause irritation: in this book, almond oil is used as the base oil for most projects using essential oils.

Anyone with a serious medical condition should not use essential oils without consulting their medical practitioner and, even then, should only use the oils with the assistance of a qualified aromatherapist. Certain essential oils should not be handled by anyone who is or may be pregnant. Of the commonly used oils, these include basil, cedarwood, chamomile (first trimester), clary sage, frankincense (first trimester), jasmine, marjoram, peppermint (first trimester) and rosemary oils.

When you first use an essential oil, it is sensible to check if your skin is sensitive to it. Do this by mixing one drop of the essential oil with a teaspoon of almond oil and then rub some into the skin of the inner arm in the same way as for the patch test. Leave for 24 hours without washing the area and, if any redness is evident, you will know that you are sensitive to the essential oil.

∞ PHOTOTOXIC OILS ∞

Most citrus oils, especially bergamot oil, make the skin more sensitive to sunlight; you should not apply them to the skin shortly before going in the sun or using a sunbed as this may cause alterations to your skin's pigmentation. It is now possible to buy citrus oils that have had the offending ingredient (bergaptene) removed but there is some question as to whether this reduces the efficacy of the oil and these treated oils are also much more expensive. Once again, one should retain a sense of proportion about this: perfumes are also phototoxic and shouldn't be worn when sunbathing, as they can cause Berloque dermatitis, an irritating skin rash.

∞ THE SAFE USE OF FRESH, ∞ NATURAL INGREDIENTS

Where a recipe calls for the inclusion of fresh, uncooked ingredients, such as fruit and eggs, it is important to use the freshest available and preferably organically grown or reared. Refrigeration is essential if the product is not used immediately and it should always be used up within the recommended period.

BELOW: The rough texture of a natural body scrub exfoliates your skin and leaves it clean and fresh.

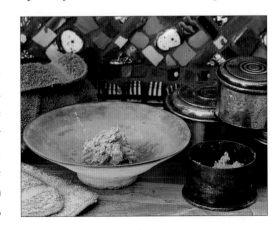

BENEFICIAL BATH OILS

72   Bath oils are an effective treatment for dry skin and, when combined with a blend of essential oils, they can strongly influence mood and health. The base oil used in these blends is almond oil, which is extremely gentle on the skin and has been combined with a smaller quantity of wheatgerm oil, which is rich in vitamin E and considered to be very good for the skin, although it shouldn't be used by anyone with a wheat sensitivity. All of the essential oils used in these blends are safe to use. They should be stored in the dark, away from heat, and the grapefruit oil should be used within six months. Similarly, the bath oils are best stored in coloured glass bottles, as exposure to light can cause the essential oil to deteriorate; plastic bottles should be avoided as the oils can react with the plastic.

The bath oils should be added to the bath after it has been run and immediately before you step into the water, or the essential oils will have evaporated into the surrounding air, instead of adhering to your skin with the carrier oil. To make the bath oils, measure the almond oil and wheatgerm oil and pour into the glass bottle. Add the essential oils and gently shake to mix. Use one tablespoon for each bath.

SEDUCTIVE ROSE AND SANDALWOOD BATH OIL

Certain essential oils have an undeniably sensuous fragrance and this is certainly true of both rose and sandalwood essential oils. Rose oil is costly to buy but it is also very powerful, so a little will go a long way. When combined with sandalwood oil, it creates a warm, spicy fragrance that will remain on the skin long after your bath.

MATERIALS
Makes about 120ml/4fl oz
100ml/3½ fl oz almond oil
20ml/4tsp wheatgerm oil
15 drops rose essential oil
10 drops sandalwood essential oil
opaque glass bottle

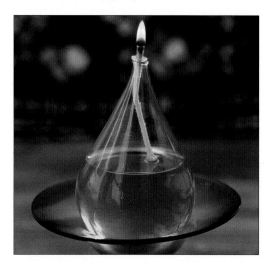

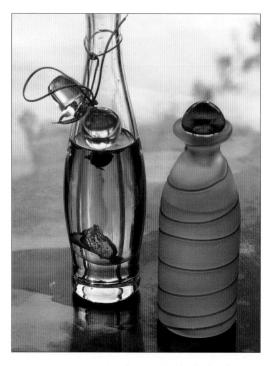

GRAPEFRUIT AND CORIANDER BATH OIL

A stimulating and refreshing combination of oils, which is a great reviver, especially when you are recovering from a cold or treating tired muscles.

MATERIALS
Makes about 120ml/4fl oz
100ml/3½ fl oz almond oil
20ml/4tsp wheatgerm oil
30 drops grapefruit essential oil
30 drops coriander essential oil
opaque glass bottle

BOTANICAL BATH SALTS

Baths scented with a mixture of salts and aromatic flowers or herbs can be formulated to relax or invigorate and also have a long tradition as a treatment for a variety of complaints. Although different salts can be used, including sodium carbonate (washing soda), magnesium sulphate (Epsom salts) or salts gathered from a therapeutic source such as the Dead Sea, the salt used in this project is simple sea salt, as some of the others can have quite powerful effects.

To use the bath salts, add two heaped tablespoons to the running water of a moderately hot bath and immerse yourself for a maximum of 15 minutes. Bath salts should not be used in very hot baths as this can elevate the heart rate too much.

Use a mortar and pestle to grind dried flowers or herbs or an electric coffee grinder. To clean the grinder, grind some oatmeal, and then grind and discard a small quantity of coffee beans.

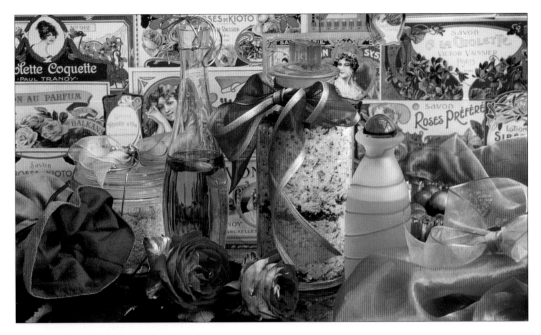

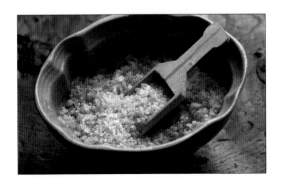

REVIVING ROSE BATH SALTS

A wonderfully aromatic mixture, this lifts the spirits and scents the skin.

~ MATERIALS ~
MAKES ABOUT 500G/1LB
10g/¼ oz dried red rose petals
mortar and pestle or electric coffee grinder
500g/1lb coarse sea salt
10 drops rose geranium essential oil
5 drops lavender essential oil
5 drops bergamot essential oil
decorative 500g/1lb glass jar, with close-fitting lid

Grind all but a handful of the rose petals. Mix the petals into the salt and add all the essential oils, stirring thoroughly. Spoon into the decorative jar, adding a decorative layer of rose petals halfway up the jar. Put the lid on firmly.

CALMING CHAMOMILE BATH SALTS

Chamomile is a widely recognized sedative; for these bath salts it has been combined with sweet marjoram, which is an effective treatment for insomnia. Be warned that these bath salts should only be used if you are planning to go to bed and sleep afterwards: sweet marjoram is an anaphrodisiac, which means that it has the opposite effect to an aphrodisiac!

~ MATERIALS ~
MAKES ABOUT 500G/1LB
500g/1lb coarse sea salt
10 drops chamomile essential oil
10 drops sweet marjoram essential oil
1–3 drops green food colouring
decorative 500g/1lb glass jar, with close-fitting lid

Combine all the ingredients and pour into the glass jar. Put the lid on firmly.

FLORAL AND HERBAL BATH BAGS

In ancient Greece and Rome, baths were scented with handfuls of flower petals or herbs; while this is still an option, they do have a tendency to clog up the plumbing. Bath bags are a practical alternative: filled with herbs or flowers and with the addition of oatmeal to soften the water, they are hung from the taps as the bath is run, releasing their fragrance into the water. You can use bath bags several times, provided that you squeeze them out after use and hang them to dry completely in a warm place.

FRAGRANT BATH BAGS

A delicious mixture of rose petals and lavender is mixed with citrus peel and bay or lemon leaves in these bath bags, which lightly scent the bath with the fragrances of summer.

—◌ *MATERIALS* ◌—
MAKES 8 BATH BAGS
8 rectangles loosely woven fabric (see above),
30 × 10cm/12 × 4in
50g/2oz dried red rose petals
50g/2oz dried lavender flowers
25g/1oz dried orange and lemon peel, cut into fine ribbons
10 g/¼ oz dried bay or lemon leaves, shredded
50g/2oz coarse oatmeal
8 fabric bags, 10 × 15cm/4 × 6in (see above)
ribbon or string

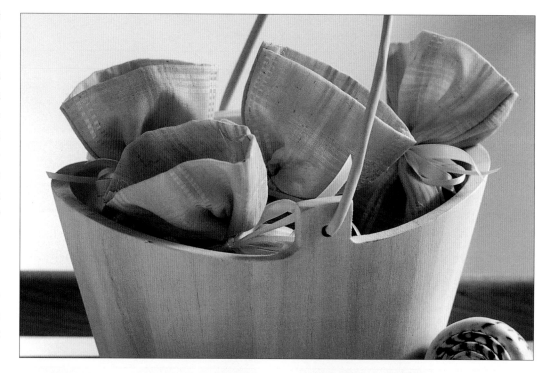

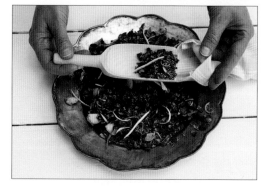

1 Fold the rectangles in half and sew up three sides. Turn right-sides out. Combine the ingredients. Fill the bags with the mixture.

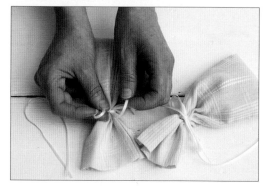

2 Tie a large loop in the ribbon or string before securing the bags, for hanging from the tap.

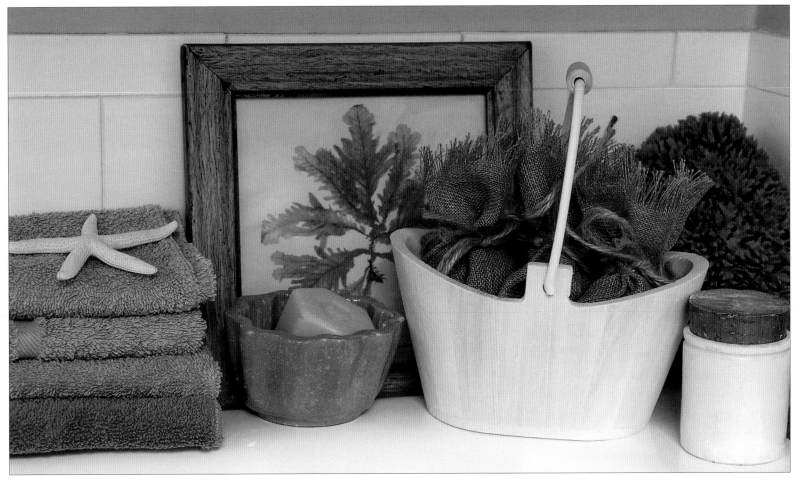

SEDATIVE BATH BAGS

A calming and sleep-inducing mixture of chamomile, lime flowers and hops has been blended with oatmeal for these bath bags, which are the perfect prelude to an early night. Make as for the Fragrant Bath Bags.

ABOVE: A complementary wooden basket holds bath bags ready for use.

RIGHT: Rose petals, lavender and orange and lemon peel are some of the ingredients of the fragrant bath bags.

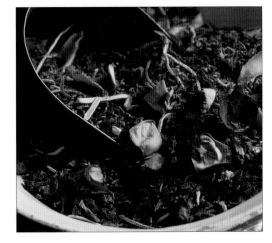

⊷ MATERIALS ⊶
MAKES 8 BATH BAGS
8 rectangles loosely woven fabric,
30 × 10cm/12 × 4in
50g/2oz chamomile flowers
50g/2oz lime flowers
25g/1oz hop flowers
50g/2oz coarse oatmeal
8 fabric bags, 10 × 15cm/4 × 6in (see above)
ribbon or string

SOAPS OF SUBSTANCE

Making soap from scratch is a lengthy and time-consuming process, involving caustic substances and chemical reactions, and is not really practical at home. However, you can add your own ingredients to simple vegetable, glycerine or olive-oil soaps and mould them into pretty shapes.

These soaps will not be as dense or as long lasting as the average bar of soap but they are nice to use as a special treat. It is important only to use these simple soaps, as the majority of manufactured soaps are difficult to work with. In both the recipes given here, finely ground nuts are added to the soaps to give them a gentle exfoliating action; they also have almond and coconut oils for richness and essential oil for fragrance. The soaps have been shaped into hearts using oiled pastry moulds in a variety of sizes; these projects make four soaps in sizes up to 7.5cm/3in.

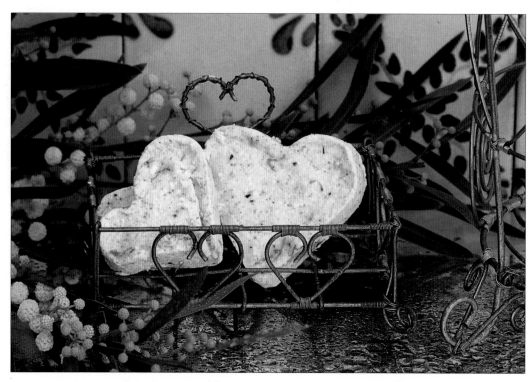

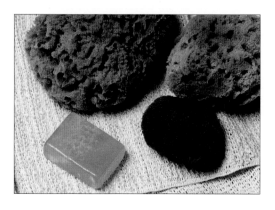

MARIGOLD AND SUNFLOWER SOAP
This sunny soap has been made from unscented vegetable glycerine soap, with added oils, ground sunflower seeds and marigold petals; it is scented with bergamot oil, which gives it a light citrus fragrance. They have been moulded in heart shapes. Make as for Olive-Oil and Lavender Soap.

LEFT: Pure soaps and natural sponges are wonderful bath companions.

—❧ *MATERIALS* ❧—
MAKES ABOUT 4 SOAPS
175g/6oz vegetable glycerine soap
grater
double boiler
25ml/1fl oz coconut oil
25ml/1fl oz almond oil
30ml/2tbsp finely ground sunflower seeds
15ml/1tbsp dried marigold petals
10 drops bergamot essential oil
spoon
heart-shaped moulds, oiled

OLIVE-OIL AND LAVENDER SOAP
Enrich a block of green Marseilles olive-oil soap with other oils and finely ground almonds and then scent it with lavender, to make pretty guest soaps. In the process an interesting, marbled effect is created.

—◦ MATERIALS ◦—
MAKES ABOUT 4 SOAPS
175g/6oz Marseilles olive-oil soap
grater
double boiler
25ml/1fl oz coconut oil
25ml/1fl oz almond oil
30ml/2tbsp ground almonds
10 drops lavender essential oil
spoon
heart-shaped moulds, oiled

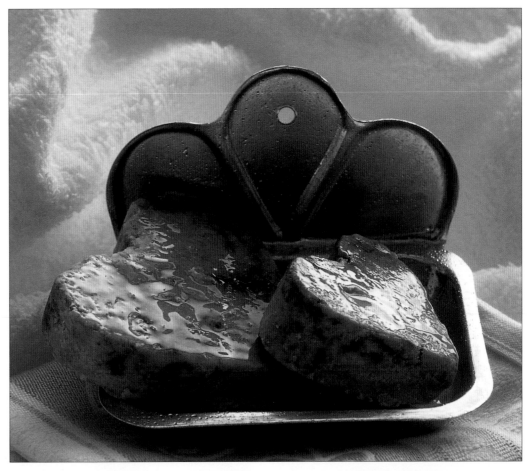

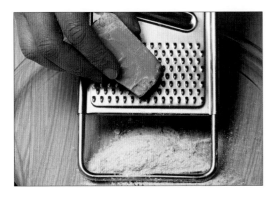

1 Grate the soap. Place the grated soap in a double boiler and leave it to soften over low heat. Add all the other ingredients.

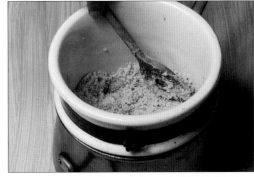

2 Stir well, until all the ingredients are evenly mixed and begin to hold together.

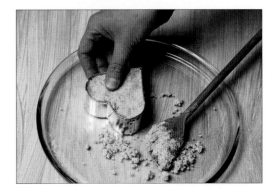

3 Press the mixture into oiled moulds and leave to set overnight. Unmould the soaps and they are ready to use.

CLASSIC CLEANSERS

78 Gentle but effective cleansers are easy to make from pure, simple ingredients. In an age when every cream and lotion seems to have added "miracle" ingredients, which promise the world and deliver disappointment, it is refreshing to discover that you can make your own creams and avoid all the hype. It is a revelation to discover how easy the basic process is: the mystique is really unwarranted. Rose water is used in both these cleansers; it has been valued for centuries as an important and effective ingredient in cosmetics.

In the Middle East, women drink rose water diluted in hot water to promote good health and beautiful skin; only use the finest rose water for this, as many of the cheaper brands are diluted and adulterated. Good quality rose waters are available by mail order.

BELOW: Store your cleanser in pretty jars so that it looks as well as feels good.

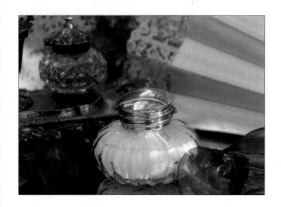

SOAPWORT CLEANSING LIQUID

This soapwort cleanser is a gentle, foaming liquid cleanser, made from the soapwort root. It is the mildest of cleansers and suitable for even the most sensitive of skins. So gentle is its cleansing action that it is also used by fabric conservators, to clean precious antique embroideries and hangings that would be damaged by even the mildest of soaps.

The soapwort root is infused in simmering water before being strained and diluted with rose water. Once made up, it will keep for a week in the bathroom or for a month in the fridge.

⇢ MATERIALS ⇠
MAKES ABOUT 600ML/1 PINT
15g/½ oz chopped soapwort root (available from herbalists)
small stainless steel or enamel saucepan
600ml/1 pint bottled spring water
unbleached paper coffee filters
50ml/2fl oz rose water
600ml/1 pint stoppered glass bottle

Place the soapwort root in the pan, with the water, bring briefly to the boil and leave to simmer gently for 15 minutes. Strain the infusion through a paper coffee filter, repeating with a clean filter if the liquid remains cloudy. Stir in the rose water and

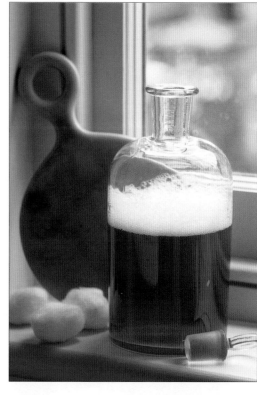

decant the mixture into the glass bottle.

To use, pour a small quantity into the palm of your hand, work to a light lather between your hands and gently massage into your face before rinsing with warm water.

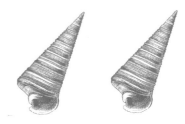

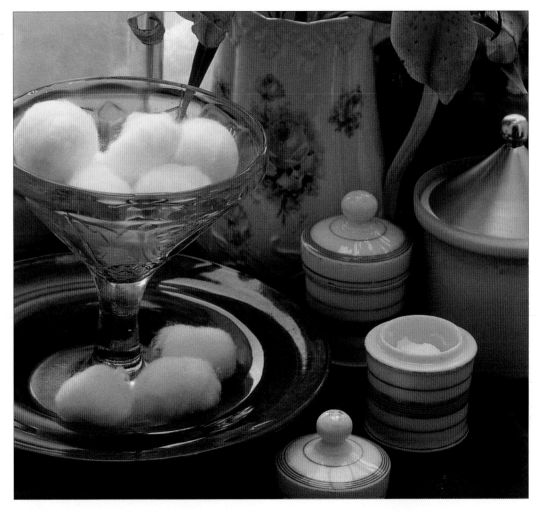

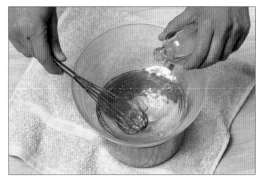

1 Melt the beeswax in a double boiler and whisk in the almond oil.

2 In a pan, add the borax to the rose water and warm gently, to dissolve. Slowly add the rose water mixture to the oils, whisking all the time. Add the essential oil, if using.

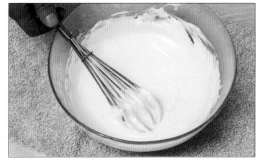

3 The mixture will quickly emulsify. Continue to whisk until the mixture has a smooth, creamy texture. Pour the cleanser into the container and leave to cool. Replace the lid securely.

To use the cleanser, smooth it on to the skin using a gentle circular movement and then remove with damp cotton wool.

ALMOND OIL CLEANSER

This almond oil cleanser is a traditional mixture of beeswax, almond oil and rose water. All creams and lotions are emulsions of oils and water and the addition of a tiny amount of borax means that this mixture emulsifies in a moment, forming a silky-smooth, creamy lotion worthy of the best cosmetic houses. Add a small amount of essential oils if you like. Rose oil is suitable for all skin types, and frankincense is particularly good for older skin.

~◎ MATERIALS ◎~
MAKES ABOUT 250ML/8FL OZ
25g/1oz white beeswax
double boiler
150ml/5fl oz almond oil
whisk
small pan
1.5ml/¼ tsp borax (available from chemists)
60ml/4tbsp rose water
2 drops rose or frankincense essential oil (optional)
250ml/8fl oz lidded, glass or ceramic jar

STIMULATING SCRUBS

⤜◈⤏

*F*ace and body scrubs are increasingly popular as part of a beauty regime. Both the gentle face scrub and citrus body scrub will efficiently exfoliate and stimulate the skin, leaving it clean and soft and ready for moisturizing. It is also a good idea to exfoliate before applying tanning lotion. Used at any time of year but especially in the dark, cold months when our bodies never see the sun, a scrub will remove dead skin and tone the skin, leaving it looking revitalized.

CITRUS BODY SCRUB

The slightly gritty texture given by ground sunflower seeds, oatmeal, sea salt and orange peel to this exfoliating scrub helps to remove dead skin cells and stimulates the blood supply to the skin, leaving you tingling and toned. The combination of the aromatic orange peel and the grapefruit oil gives it a fresh scent.

⤜◈ *MATERIALS* ◈⤏
MAKES ENOUGH FOR 5 TREATMENTS
45ml/3tbsp freshly ground sunflower seeds
45ml/3tbsp medium oatmeal
45ml/3tbsp flaked sea salt
45ml/3tbsp finely grated orange peel
3 drops grapefruit essential oil
lidded glass jar
almond oil

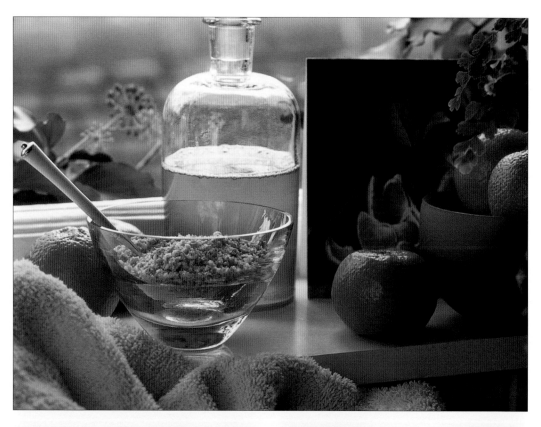

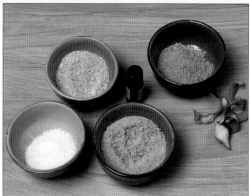

1 Thoroughly mix all the ingredients and store in a sealed glass jar.

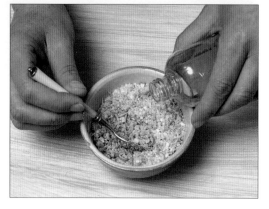

2 Mix to a paste with almond oil before using. Rub over the body, paying particular attention to areas of hard, dry skin such as the elbows, knees and ankles. Remove the residue before showering or bathing.

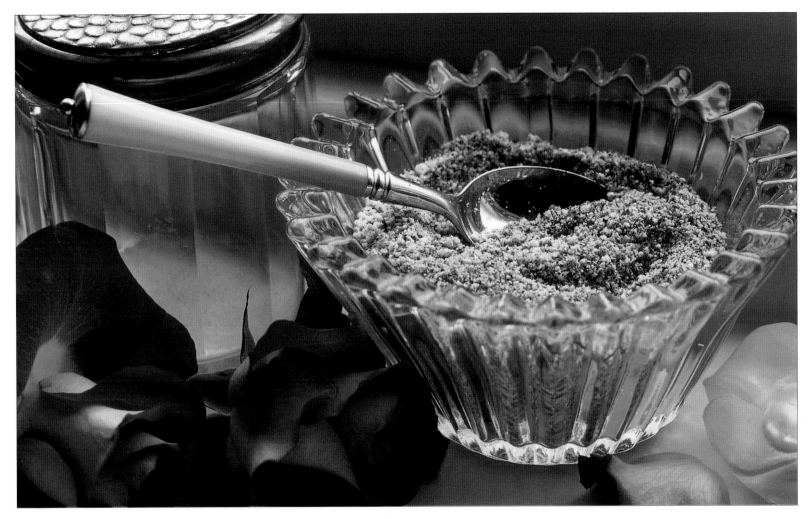

GENTLE FACE SCRUB

This is a face scrub worthy of Cleopatra, with its luxurious blend of almonds, oatmeal, milk and rose petals. The rose petals should be bought from an herbalist or, if you want to use petals from your garden, be sure that they have not been sprayed with chemicals. The rose petals can be powdered in a pestle and mortar or in an electric coffee grinder. When mixed with almond oil, the scrub will cleanse the face and leave it silky-soft.

⊸ MATERIALS ⊶
MAKES ENOUGH FOR 10 TREATMENTS
45ml/3tbsp ground almonds (without skin)
45ml/3tbsp medium oatmeal
45ml/3tbsp powdered milk
30ml/2tbsp powdered rose petals
mixing bowl
spoon
lidded glass jar
almond oil

Mix all the ingredients together and store in a sealed glass jar. Before using, mix to a soft paste with almond oil. With the lightest of touches, gently rub it into the skin, using a circular motion and being careful to avoid the delicate area around the eyes. Rinse off with warm water and pat your face dry.

FACE PACKS

There is an enjoyably ritualistic feeling to smearing a face pack over the skin and leaving it to dry, almost as if you were returning to the ancient rites of our ancestors. In some ways, we are: the beneficial effects of clay and oatmeal on the skin have been known for centuries, and there are records of face packs being used to treat blemished skin as far back as in Ancient Egypt.

PAPAYA FACE PACK
The papaya fruit contains a powerful enzyme that digests dead skin and is therefore a valuable constituent of this face pack. Here, it is combined with soothing aloe vera juice and green clay to make a gentle but effective face pack. Green clay is a very fine clay, available from specialists; aloe vera juice can be obtained from healthfood shops and chemists (drugstores).

─◦ MATERIALS ◦─
MAKES ENOUGH FOR 3 TREATMENTS
¼ medium-sized papaya
blender or food processor
7ml/1½ tsp aloe vera juice
small bowl
spoon
60ml/4tbsp green clay
small glass jar, with rubber seal

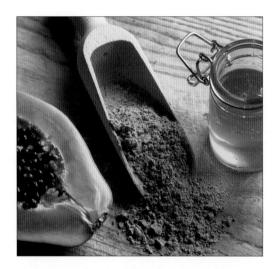

Peel the papaya and blend it till smooth. Add the aloe vera juice and blend again. Pour the mixture into a small bowl and slowly stir in the clay to form a smooth paste. Spoon into the glass jar and use immediately, or put the lid on firmly and store in the fridge for up to five days.

To use the papaya face pack, spread it over your face, avoiding the delicate eye area, and leave it for 20 minutes. Rinse off with cool water and then splash your face with cold water before patting it dry.

> ### WARNING
> Carry out a patch test before using the face pack (see The Safe Use of Natural Products).

GENTLE OATMEAL MASK
Very sensitive skin can find a face mask that contains clay slightly irritating; if this is you, this gentlest of face masks is the answer. A creamy mix of oatmeal, egg and honey soothes and nourishes the skin, while gently lifting impurities from it.

─◦ MATERIALS ◦─
MAKES ENOUGH FOR 1 TREATMENT
15ml/1tbsp runny honey
1 egg yolk
small bowl
spoon
up to 60ml/4tbsp fine oatmeal

Mix the honey and egg yolk together and then slowly stir in sufficient oatmeal to make a soft paste. Use immediately.

To use, smooth the mask on to the skin and leave for 15 minutes. Rinse off with lukewarm water and pat dry.

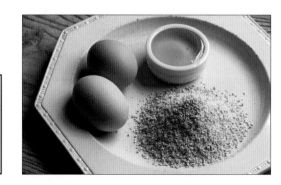

Aromatic Massage Oils

Gentle-but-firm massage is a wonderful reviver of tired, tender or tense muscles, especially when the aches are smoothed away with a fragrant oil. A massage oil is a blend of a base oil with a very small quantity of essential oils. With very few exceptions, essential oils should never be used undiluted on the skin and, if the massage oil is to be used on babies or children, the amount of essential oils in these recipes should be halved.

The base for these massage oils is a blend of almond oil with a small quantity of wheatgerm oil. If you have a sensitivity to wheat, you should omit the wheatgerm oil and add more almond oil.

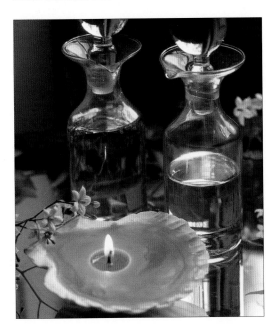

Soothing Massage Oil

A pleasant blend of lavender, clary sage and chamomile oils is ideal when you want to soothe away stress and help relieve tense, nervous headaches. When a full massage is not possible, try gently massaging in a couple of drops of the oil behind the ears, using a circular motion.

Although generally safe to use, clary sage and chamomile oils should be avoided during pregnancy.

⋙ MATERIALS ⋘
Makes 50ml/2fl oz
45ml/3tbsp almond oil
1.5ml/¼ tsp wheatgerm oil
glass bottle, with stopper
10 drops lavender essential oil
5 drops clary sage essential oil
5 drops chamomile essential oil

Pour the almond and wheatgerm oils into the glass bottle, add the essential oils and gently shake to mix. Store the bottle in a cool, dark place.

> **WARNING**
> Before using any oils for massage, carry out a patch test (see The Safe Use of Natural Products).

Seductive Massage Oil

A number of essential oils are reputed to have aphrodisiac qualities and, while this is hard to prove, it is certainly true that certain fragrances seem more sensuous than others. Among these, rose, jasmine, neroli and ylang-ylang are considered the finest and, inevitably, are also among the most expensive oils. The rose oil which is available in the shops is generally diluted with jojoba oil, to make it less expensive, but its fragrance is barely perceptible compared with the intense fragrance of rose otto (also known as attar) or rose absolute, which are two types of pure rose oil. To obtain either of these, order them by mail order from a specialist; if the scent of roses is a particular favourite, this would be a worthwhile purchase. Rose geranium essential oil is a cheaper alternative to rose oil.

⋙ MATERIALS ⋘
Makes enough for 3 Full-body Massages or
6 Neck and Shoulder Massages
50ml/2fl oz almond oil
1.5ml/¼ tsp wheatgerm oil
glass bottle, with stopper
15 drops rose essential oil
5 drops coriander essential oil
2 drops cedarwood essential oil

Make as for Soothing Massage Oil.

TRADITIONAL COLD CREAM

Long before the days of complicated skin cream formulations enriched with all sorts of magical ingredients, women relied on a simple cold cream, made from pure, natural ingredients to moisturize their skins. In spite of cosmetic-company hype, scientists tell us that there is very little difference between the hugely expensive creams and the cheapest and that all will have a similar effect, provided that they are used regularly on clean skin and are made from quality ingredients.

This traditional, rose-scented cold cream has a pleasant, light texture, which makes it easy to use and ensures that it is quickly absorbed by the skin, leaving it feeling soft and pampered. Do not use on broken skin.

--- ❧ MATERIALS ❧ ---
MAKES ABOUT 300ML/½ PINT
50g/2oz white beeswax
double boiler or bowl
whisk
120ml/4fl oz almond oil
50ml/2fl oz rose water
small pan
2.5ml/½ tsp borax
spoon
120ml/4fl oz bottled spring water, heated
4 drops rose essential oil (optional)
300ml/½ pint lidded glass or ceramic jar

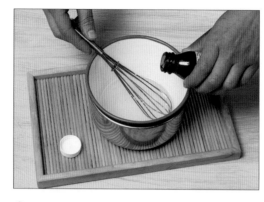

1 Put the beeswax in a double boiler or in a bowl over a pan of water and heat gently until it is melted. Off the heat, slowly whisk in the almond oil.

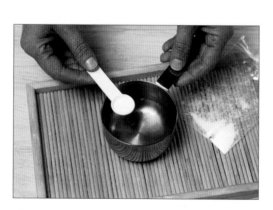

2 Gently warm the rose water in a small pan and add the borax. Stir until the borax has dissolved. Add the rose water mixture to the hot water.

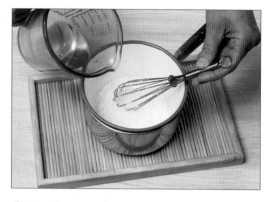

3 Slowly pour the water and rose water mixture into the melted wax and oil, whisking all the time. As the water is added, the mixture will start to emulsify, turning white and creamy.

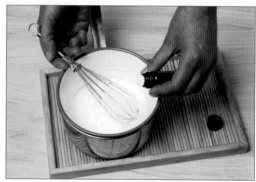

4 Keep whisking as the mixture cools, to ensure an even texture. Add the rose oil at this stage, if using. Spoon the cold cream into the jar and seal when it has cooled.

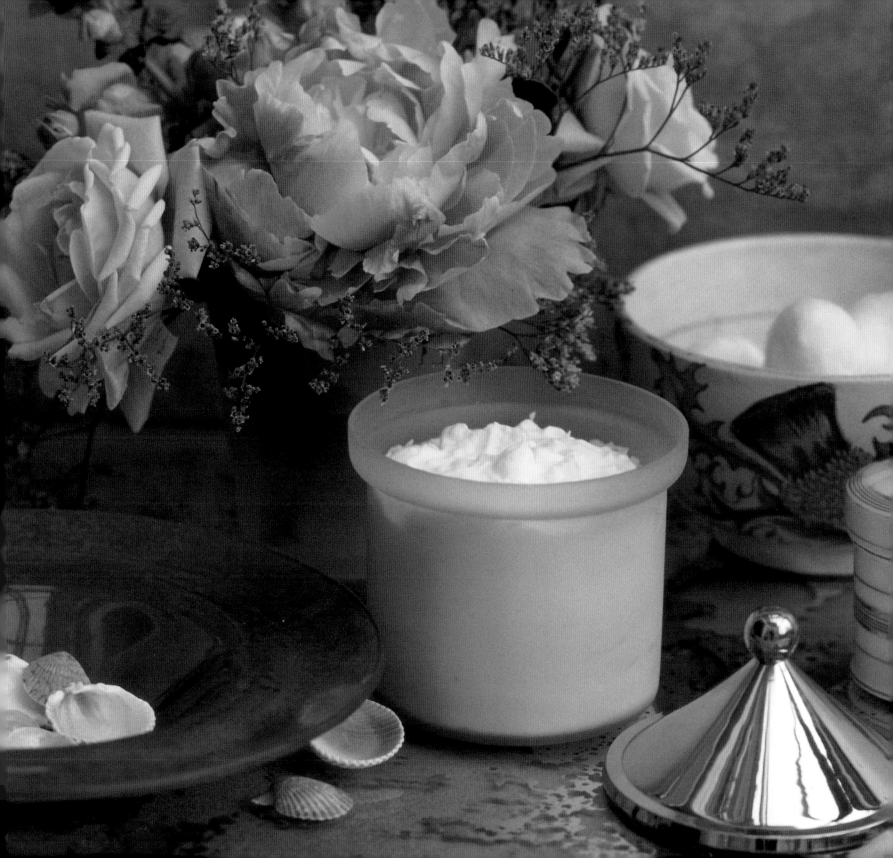

LUXURIOUS BODY LOTIONS

We don't always have the time or the inclination to make beauty preparations from scratch but, if you start with a basic, unscented, ready-made product, you can add your own fragrance and use decorative containers to make something luxurious. These beautifully presented body lotions would make wonderful presents, if you could bear to give them away. Alternatively, enjoy them yourself for pure pampering pleasure.

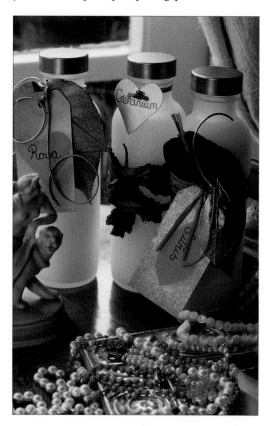

ROSE BODY LOTION

A fragrant lotion, reminiscent of high summer and romance. Rose oil is excellent for all skin types. The frosted glass bottle has been decorated with gilded rose leaves and a gold label with a heart motif.

☙ MATERIALS ❧
MAKES 175ML/6FL OZ
175ml/6fl oz unscented body lotion
10 drops rose essential oil
decorative, screw-topped bottle

Mix the body lotion and rose oil together and pour into a bottle with a tight lid.

GERANIUM BODY LOTION

A spicily fragrant lotion which is pleasantly aromatic. Geranium oil is derived from a relative of the scented leaf geranium and the fragrance is very like that of the crushed leaves. The bottle has been decorated with a geranium leaf and a gilded, heart-shaped label.

☙ MATERIALS ❧
MAKES 175ML/6FL OZ
175ml/6fl oz unscented body lotion
15 drops geranium essential oil
bottle

Make as for Rose Body Lotion.

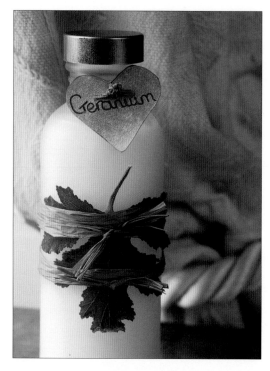

CITRUS BODY LOTION

A refreshing blend of grapefruit and bergamot oils give this body lotion a delightful, light fragrance. Citrus oils have a short shelf-life and should be used within six months of purchase. As many of them, including bergamot, are phototoxic, they should not be applied to the skin before going into the sun or using a sunbed. The bottle has been decorated with a lemon leaf and a gilded label.

☙ MATERIALS ❧
MAKES 175ML/6FL OZ
175ml/6fl oz unscented body lotion
10 drops grapefruit essential oil
5 drops bergamot essential oil

Make as for Rose Body Lotion.

HAND AND FOOT CREAMS

As with the body lotions, these hand and foot creams are made very simply by adding suitable essential oils to an unscented cream. Look for a lanolin-rich cream or one that includes cocoa butter, as both hands and feet benefit from something with a richer formulation. Although most creams and lotions are best stored in glass or ceramic containers, in this case it is sensible and practical to keep the lotion in a pump-action plastic bottle (below), which makes it so much easier to use.

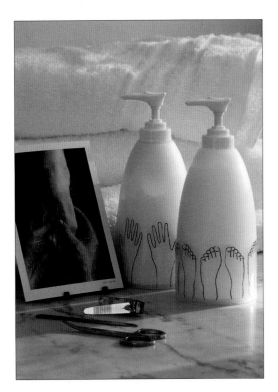

TI-TREE FOOT CREAM

While our hands tend to suffer from damage caused from overuse and abuse, our feet are more likely to suffer from neglect. We take them utterly for granted, yet seldom pamper and care for them the way we do the rest of the body; this is a shame, because well-cared-for feet look and feel so much better. Ti-tree is one of the best essential oils to incorporate in a foot cream. It has healing, antiseptic properties and also has a fungicidal action, which will protect the feet from the various unpleasant foot complaints which can be picked up at the pool or gym.

◦ MATERIALS ◦
MAKES 120ML/4FL OZ
120ml/4fl oz unscented hand cream
15 drops ti-tree essential oil
bowl
spoon
pump-action plastic bottle
funnel

Blend the essential oils thoroughly into the unscented hand cream and pour into the plastic bottle through a funnel.

> **WARNING**
> Lemon oil is phototoxic.

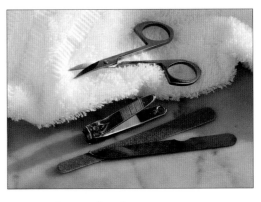

ABOVE: A basic nailcare kit.

HEALING HAND CREAM

The oils in this cream are good for the hands: the chamomile soothes, the geranium helps heal cuts and the lemon oil softens skin.

◦ MATERIALS ◦
MAKES 120ML/4FL OZ
10 drops chamomile essential oil
5 drops geranium essential oil
5 drops lemon essential oil
120ml/4fl oz unscented hand cream
bowl
spoon
pump-action plastic bottle
funnel

Blend the essential oils thoroughly into the unscented hand cream and pour into the plastic bottle through a funnel.

REFRESHING COLOGNE AND FRAGRANT PERFUME

88   W e have been scenting our bodies since our ancestors first discovered fragrant herbs, spices, gums and resins. Scent is an important ingredient in the chemistry of attraction and most of us do not feel fully clothed unless we are wearing a favourite perfume. Colognes and perfumes are easily made at home, using vodka as the base, and, although they will not have the strength or the lasting power of commercial varieties, they are still deliciously fragrant and pleasant to use. Although not essential, the addition of a fixative tincture to both cologne and perfume will help the fragrance to last longer.

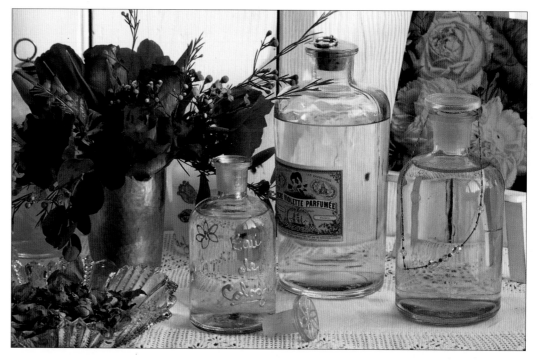

SUMMER SCENT

A delicate blend of rose, geranium and bergamot create a prettily scented *eau de parfum* reminiscent of summer gardens.

~ MATERIALS ~
MAKES ABOUT 120ML/4FL OZ
100ml/3½ fl oz vodka
glass bottle with stopper, sterilized
10 drops rose essential oil
10 drops geranium essential oil
30 drops bergamot essential oil
15ml/1tbsp distilled water
2.5ml/½ tsp fixative tincture (optional; see above)
unbleached paper coffee filters
decorative bottle or jar, with tightly fitting lid

Measure the vodka into the bottle. Add the essential oils. Stopper the bottle, gently shake to mix and leave to stand for 48 hours. Add the distilled water and fixative, if using. Replace the stopper, gently shake to mix and leave to stand for one week. Shake the bottle and then strain through coffee filter papers, until the *eau de parfum* is clear and sparkling. Store as above.

> **WARNING**
> Bergamot oil is phototoxic.

> *TO MAKE FIXATIVE TINCTURE*
> Mix 5ml/1tsp of powdered gum benzoin or orris root with 30ml/2tbsp of vodka. Pour into a small, screw-topped bottle and shake vigorously, to mix. Leave to stand for at least 24 hours; longer is better. To use, pour off without disturbing the residue. Gum benzoin and orris root are available from companies selling pot-pourri ingredients and from herbalists.

EAU DE COLOGNE

Eau de Cologne was first made in 1709 by an Italian barber living in Germany; it consisted of grape spirits and oils of neroli, lavender, rosemary and bergamot. It was once even taken internally, as a supposed cure-all for humans and animals alike. The fragrance of *eau de Cologne* is light and refreshing and it is perfect as an after-bath body splash; or keep it in an aerosol bottle in the fridge in hot weather and use as a scented cooling spray.

~ MATERIALS ~
MAKES ABOUT 150ML/¼ PINT
120ml/4fl oz vodka
funnel, sterilized
glass jar with stopper, sterilized
20 drops sweet orange essential oil
10 drops bergamot essential oil
10 drops lavender essential oil
2 drops rosemary essential oil
50ml/2fl oz distilled water
5ml/1tsp fixative tincture (optional)
unbleached paper coffee filters
decorative bottle or jar, with tightly fitting lid

WARNING
Sweet orange oil and bergamot oil are
phototoxic.

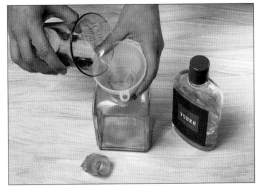

1 Measure the vodka into the sterile jar.

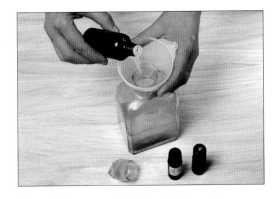

2 Add the essential oils. Replace the stopper, gently shake to mix and leave to stand for 48 hours.

3 Add the distilled water and fixative, if using. Replace the stopper, gently shake to mix and leave to stand for one week.

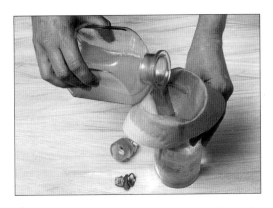

4 Shake the bottle and then strain through a series of filter papers, until the cologne is clear and sparkling. Store in a decorative bottle or jar, making sure the lid seals well.

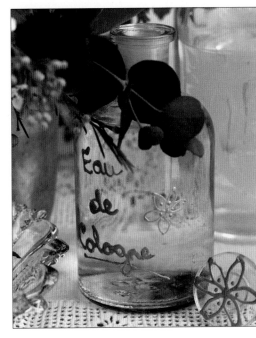

GENTLE EYE TREATMENTS

The skin around the eyes is the most delicate on the face and also the first to look in need of attention if we are tired or stressed. There are a number of simple treatments for tired eyes, which, when combined with gentle moisturizing, will revive and revitalize. All these treatments involve lying down with your eyes covered for at least 15 minutes, and this enforced relaxing is probably almost as important a part of the treatment as the compresses.

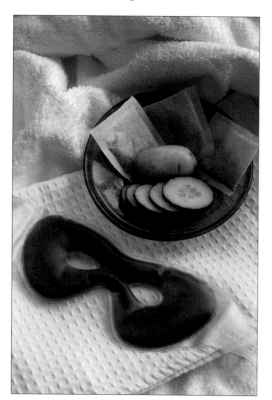

TEA-BAG TREATMENT

Tea contains tannin, which is astringent and will firm the skin. Place a couple of ordinary Indian tea-bags on a saucer and pour hot water over them. Cover with another saucer and stand in the fridge to cool. Gently squeeze the excess moisture from the tea-bags and lie down with them covering your eyes for 10–15 minutes. Remove the tea-bags and gently pat the skin dry before dabbing on moisturizing lotion.

COOLING CUCUMBER

This is the simplest treatment of all. Place a slice of cucumber over each eye while you relax for 15 minutes. The cucumber will very gently tone the skin around the eyes and help restore tired eyes.

POTATO PAMPERING

An old country remedy for tired skin around the eyes is to grate potato finely and place it between two layers of muslin before applying it as a compress over the eyes. Certainly, the starch in the potatoes seems to tighten the skin, so it may be more than an old wives' tale.

LEFT: Revive tired eyes with tea, potatoes or cucumber, and a long rest.

CHAMOMILE COMPRESSES

This is a tried and tested treatment for tired eyes. Although it can be done using herbal tea-bags, if you have time, it is worth making the compresses from muslin and whole chamomile flowers rather than the more powdery mix that often goes into tea-bags. As with the tea-bags, cover them with hot water and then leave them to cool in the fridge before lying down for 20 minutes with the compresses over the eyes.

MATERIALS
FOR EACH COMPRESS
double-thickness 15cm/6in square unbleached muslin
scissors
5g/⅛ oz/good handful dried chamomile flowers
20cm/8in fine ribbon or string

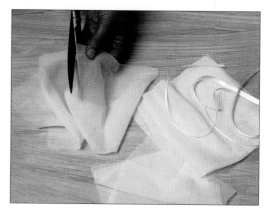

1 Cut the muslin into the required number of squares.

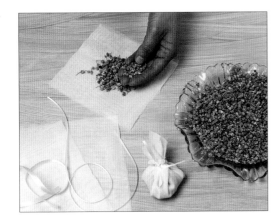

2 Place a handful of chamomile flowers in the centre of the muslin square.

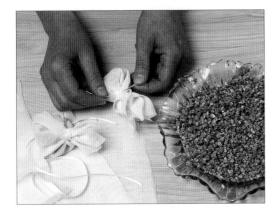

3 Gather the muslin into a bundle and tie it with ribbon or string.

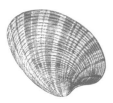
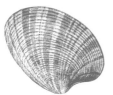

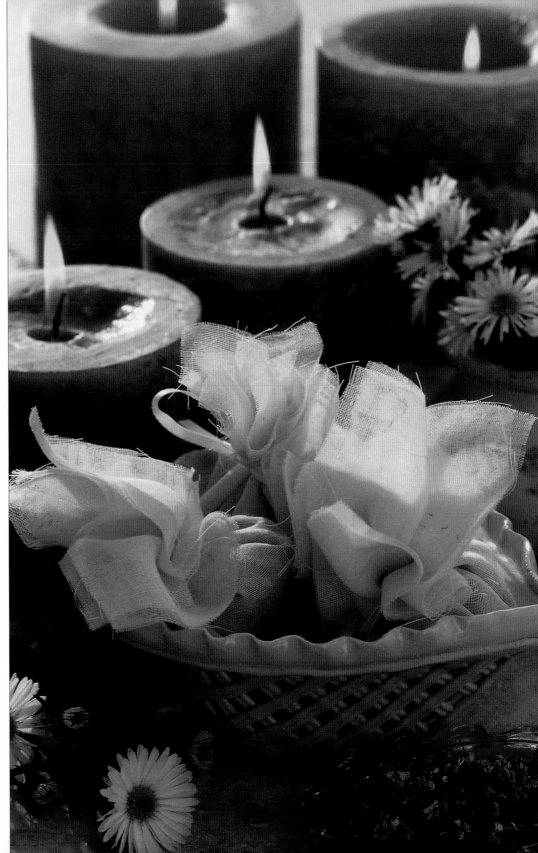

DELICIOUS DUSTING POWDER

*T*here is a tendency to think of dusting powders as being the province of just bathed babies and elderly ladies, but this needn't be so. A talcum powder, dusted all over the body, is a wonderful way to coat the body with fragrance.

Dusting powders can be made from scratch or you can use unscented talc as a base. Either way you will be able to formulate a scented powder quite different from the commercial talcum powders. Dusting powders look wonderful in shallow bowls accompanied by a pretty powder puff; alternatively, a sugar-shaker makes them easy to use.

SINGLE FRAGRANCE DUSTING POWDERS

These dusting powders are the simplest of all to make, especially if your base is a ready-made unscented talcum powder. For every 5 tablespoons of talc you will need I tablespoon of cornflour, scented with 5 drops of your favourite essential oil. Fragrance is so personal that you will need to decide for yourself the properties of the different oils, but it is generally accepted that jasmine sets the scene for seduction, roses are romantic and peppermint or lemon are good to use after vigorous exercise at the gym.

LUSCIOUS LAVENDER BODY POWDER

A soft blend of lavender, coriander and geranium with a hint of fresh lemon gives this body powder a delightful fragrance. Use it after your evening bath. In Ancient Egypt, high-ranking nobles and officials would sleep in beds scented with fragrant powders, believing that the fragrance was better absorbed by the skin and more long lasting.

MATERIALS
MAKES ABOUT 150G/5OZ
60ml/4tbsp white kaolin clay
(available from pharmacies)
60ml/4tbsp arrowroot
60ml/4tbsp cornflour or 180ml/12tbsp
unscented talc
15ml/1tbsp cornflour (cornstarch)
3 drops lavender essential oil
3 drops coriander essential oil
3 drops lemon essential oil
3 drops geranium essential oil
decorative, lidded container

In a deep bowl, mix together the clay and arrowroot and add the cornflour (cornstarch) or unscented talc. Put the 15ml/1tbsp of cornflour into a separate small bowl and add the essential oils. Stir thoroughly. Add the scented cornflour to the larger bowl and mix. Decant into the container.

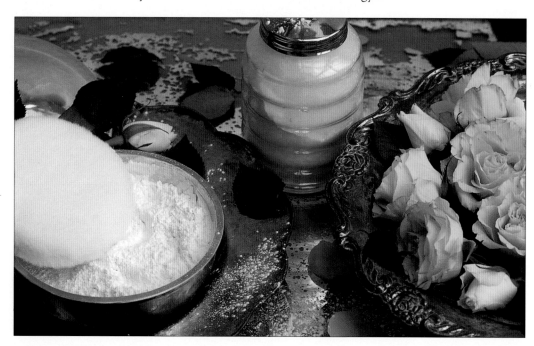

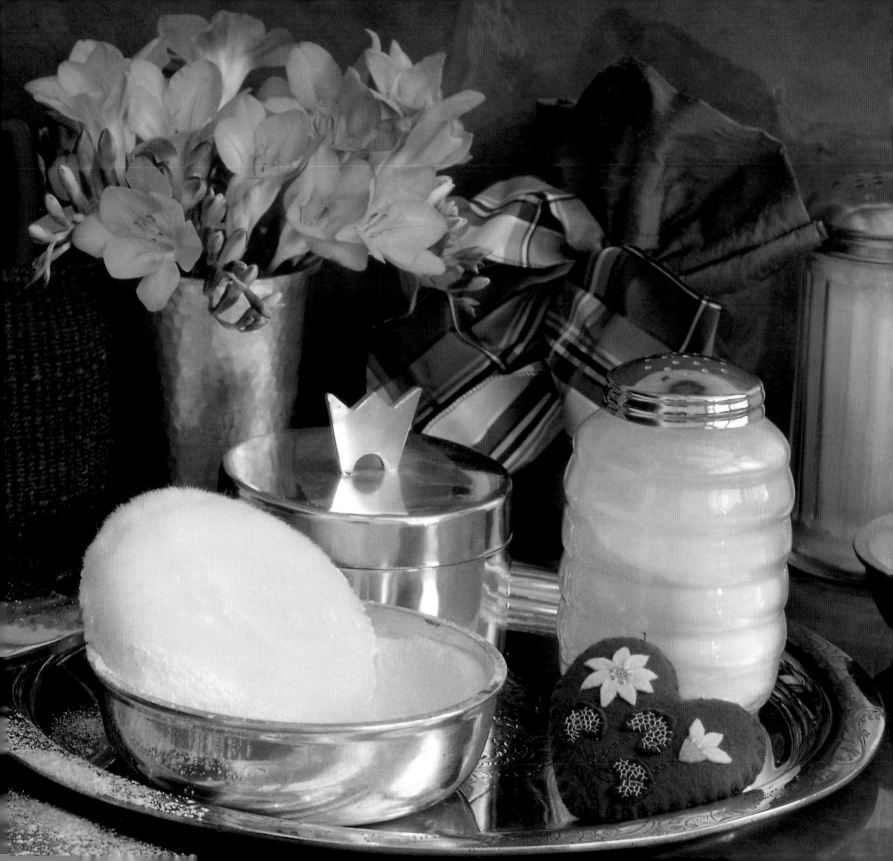

HEALTHY HAIR

*A*nyone perusing the hair-care shelves at the supermarket or chemist (drugstore) will know that, nowadays, there is a bewildering range of products for every type of hair. These highly sophisticated products can make your hair look wonderful, but so can far simpler treatments, which have been tried and trusted over hundreds of years. Good hairdressers do recommend a varied programme of hair care, because consistently using any one product can lead to build-up on hair and scalp. These herbal hair rinses and other treatments use natural ingredients to leave your hair in really good condition.

FAIR-HAIR RINSE

Chamomile and rosemary have been combined with cider vinegar and used in hair rinses for hundreds of years. The herbs enhance hair colour and the vinegar is a wonderful scalp conditioner.

Chamomile has long been favoured by blondes for their fair hair; although it does not bleach it enhances the natural colour.

✦ MATERIALS ✦

MAKES ENOUGH FOR 3 TREATMENTS
50g/2oz dried chamomile flowers
wide-necked glass jar, with rubber seal
a piece of muslin or paper coffee filters
50ml/2fl oz cider vinegar
5 drops chamomile essential oil
glass bottle, with stopper

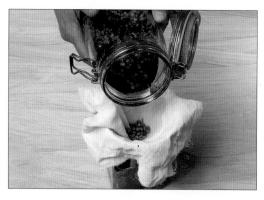

2 Seal the jar and leave to stand overnight. Strain the infusion through muslin or paper filters, until it is clear.

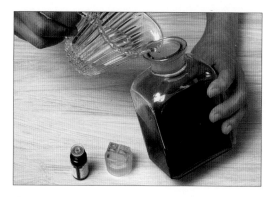

3 Add the cider vinegar and essential oil. Store in a stoppered glass bottle in the fridge and use within one week, as a final rinse when washing your hair.

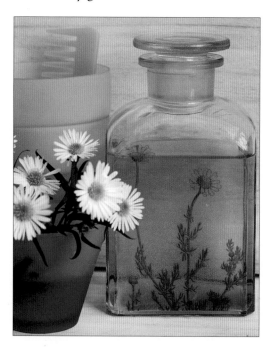

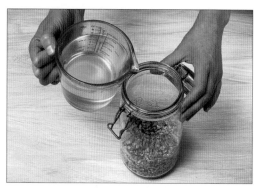

1 Measure the chamomile flowers into the wide-necked jar and pour 900ml/1½ pints of just-boiled water on to the flowers.

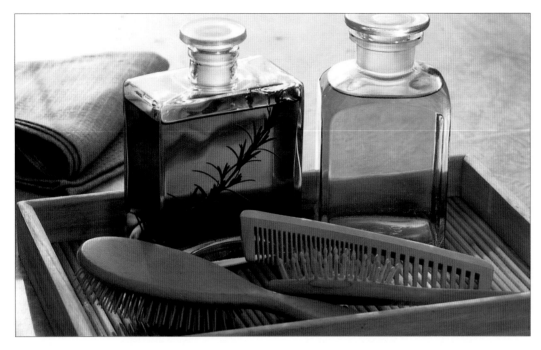

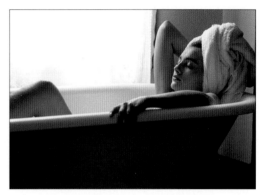

DARK-HAIR RINSE

This rinse uses the same basic ingredients as the fair-hair rinse but substitutes sprigs of fresh rosemary and rosemary oil for the chamomile flowers and oil.

-❧ MATERIALS ❧-
MAKES ENOUGH FOR 1 TREATMENT
50g/2oz fresh rosemary sprigs
wide-necked glass jar with rubber seal
muslin or paper coffee filters
50ml/2fl oz cider vinegar
5 drops rosemary essential oil
glass bottle, with stopper

Make as for the Fair-Hair Rinse.

> *WARNING*
> Pregnant women should omit the rosemary essential oil.

HAIR RESCUER

A rich nourishing formula, to help improve the condition of dry and damaged hair.

-❧ MATERIALS ❧-
MAKES ENOUGH FOR 1 TREATMENT
30ml/2tbsp olive oil
30ml/2tbsp light sesame oil
2 eggs
30ml/2tbsp coconut milk
30ml/2tbsp runny honey
5ml/1tsp coconut oil
blender or food processor

Whizz all the ingredients together in the blender or food processor, until smooth. Transfer to a bottle. Use within three days and keep refrigerated.

To use, after shampooing, comb the mixture through your hair. Leave for 5 minutes and then rinse with warm water.

WARM-OIL TREATMENT

Use this treatment once a month to improve the hair texture and condition the scalp.

-❧ MATERIALS ❧-
MAKES ENOUGH FOR 5 TREATMENTS
90ml/6tbsp coconut oil
3 drops rosemary essential oil
2 drops ti-tree essential oil
2 drops lavender essential oil
dark-coloured glass bottle, with stopper

Pour all the ingredients into the bottle and shake gently to mix.

Use the oil sparingly on dry hair; the head should not be saturated. Massage it in before covering your head with a hot towel for 20 minutes. Shampoo as normal.

Aromatic Bubble Bath

◈

*B*ubble baths are wonderfully frivolous things; fragrant and foamy, they are the perfect setting for a bit of pleasant self-indulgence. Although there are some existing recipes for making bubble bath from a blend of soap flakes and other ingredients, they don't seem to work very well: the bubbles are rather half-hearted and disappear before you can get in the bath. Unscented liquid soap or clear shampoo is a good base ingredient, which can be scented and coloured to give the desired result.

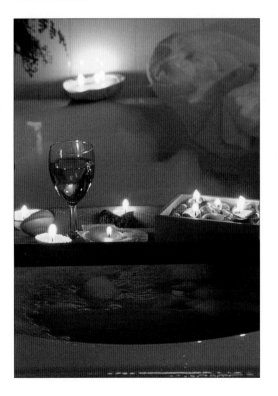

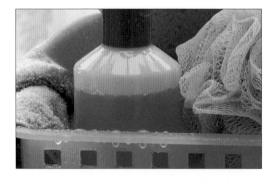

GRAPEFRUIT AND GINGER BUBBLES
The fresh, zesty fragrance of grapefruit combined with stimulating ginger make this an ideal mixture for a refreshing bath. The addition of glycerine will help soften the skin and counter the effect of hard water. Depending on how many bubbles you want, squeeze a tablespoon or more into the stream of water as you run the bath.

⊸ *MATERIALS* ⊷
MAKES 150ML/¼ PINT
120ml/4fl oz unscented liquid soap
25ml/1fl oz glycerine from a chemist (drugstore)
1 drop green food colouring (optional)
35 drops grapefruit essential oil
15 drops ginger essential oil
squeezable plastic bottle

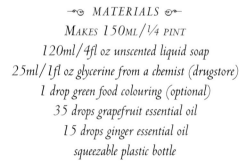

LEFT: Bubble bath, candlelight and wine transform your bathroom into a place of sybaritic indulgence.

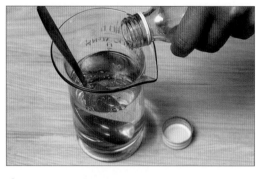

1 Mix the glycerine into the liquid soap.

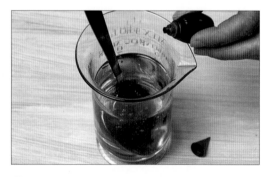

2 Stir in the food colouring, if using.

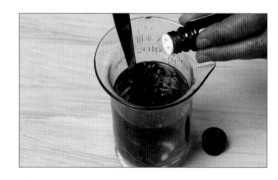

3 Add the essential oils and stir thoroughly. Store in a squeezable bottle.

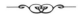

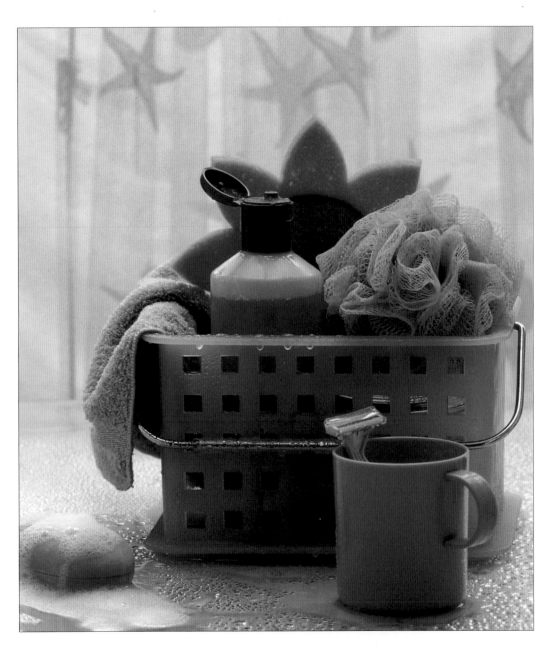

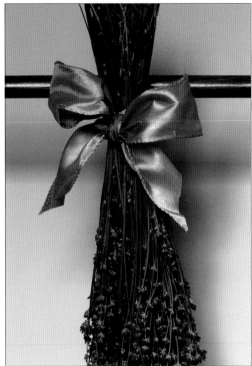

ABOVE: Hang a bunch of lavender in your bathroom.

LAVENDER BUBBLE BATH

The perfect relaxing bath after a stressful day: lavender helps relieve tense, nervous headaches.

—◦ *MATERIALS* ◦—
medium-sized bottle of clear, unscented shampoo
45ml/3tbsp dried lavender flowers
5 drops lavender essential oil
wide-necked, screw-topped glass jar
fine sieve
squeezable plastic bottle

Place all the ingredients in the glass jar, replace the lid and shake to mix. Leave to stand in a warm place for two weeks, shaking the jar occasionally. Strain the liquid and pour into a plastic bottle.

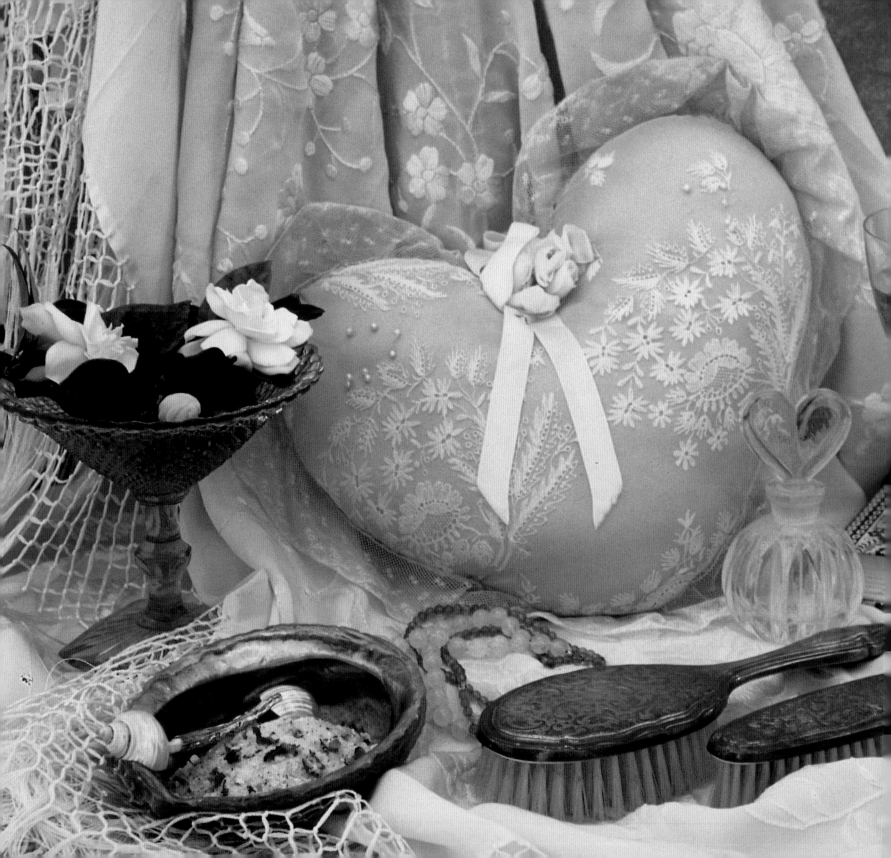

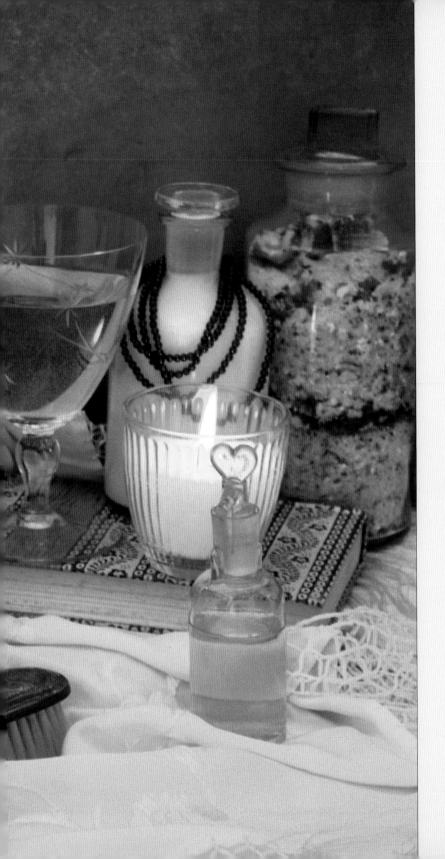

Chapter Four

PAMPERING

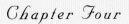

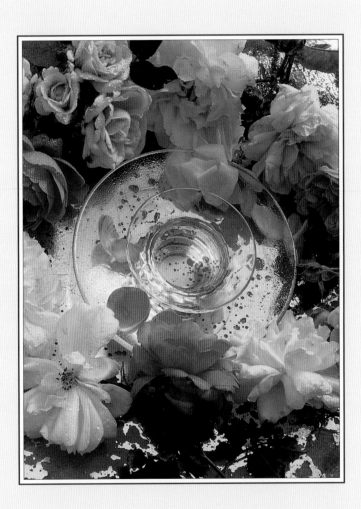

ABOVE: Massage oils scented with essential flower oils are a sensual delight.

LEFT: The first step towards pampering your body is to surround yourself

with pretty things.

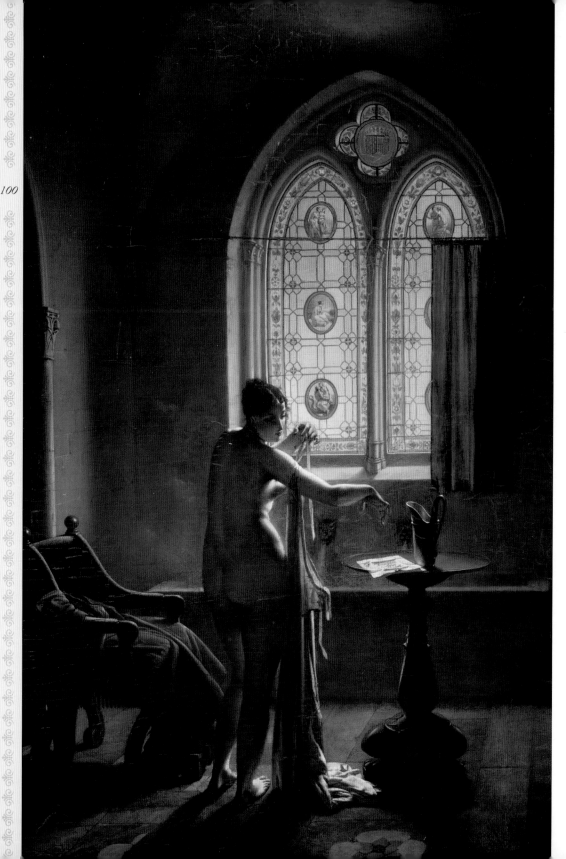

Now that you have created your own personal oasis in the bathroom and filled it with lotions, oils and creams made from luscious natural ingredients, it is time to pamper your body and take time out for yourself.

The pleasures of the bath and bathing are available to everyone, even those with neither the time nor the inclination to redecorate the bathroom or make their own lotions and potions. A personal oasis is as much a state of mind as a customized room. The key to enjoying these pleasures is the decision to take time to enjoy the experience of bathing and its accompanying rituals. The bathroom and its rituals, if unhurried, will accomplish far more than cleansing the body and softening the skin.

～ LEARNING TO RELAX ～

In theory, we understand that it is important to relax but how often do we really do so? It is always last on the list of our priorities; even when we do sit down, we find it hard to "switch off" properly. Before we know it, we are off across the room to carry out some task that has caught our attention and relaxing is forgotten. We need to learn to take time for ourselves, to recharge our batteries and

LEFT: The unselfconscious grace of this woman as she undresses shows a woman who is at ease with her body. Nowadays we are often obsessed with trying to be something we are not rather than enjoying who we are.

understand that this is an essential part of a healthy life, not a selfish indulgence! Taking half an hour for yourself in the bathroom is a good starting point. It is more difficult to be distracted when you are naked and up to your neck in water and, if the bath is sweetly

RIGHT: *Slowly massaging cream into the skin is relaxing as well as moisturizing.*

BELOW: *With the advent of advertising women were used to present idealised images.*

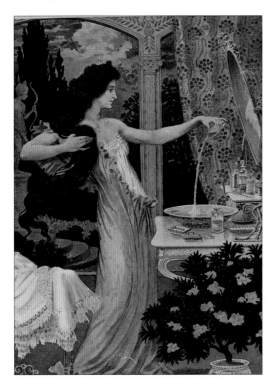

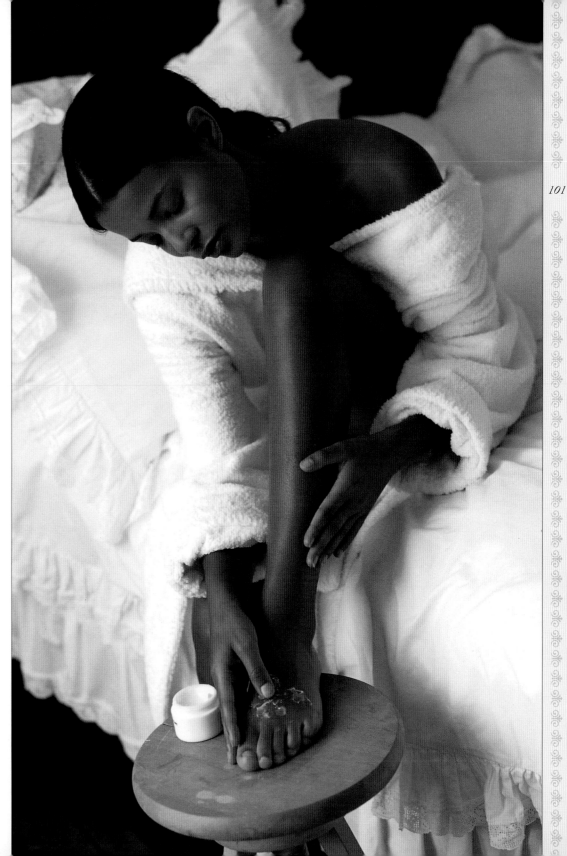

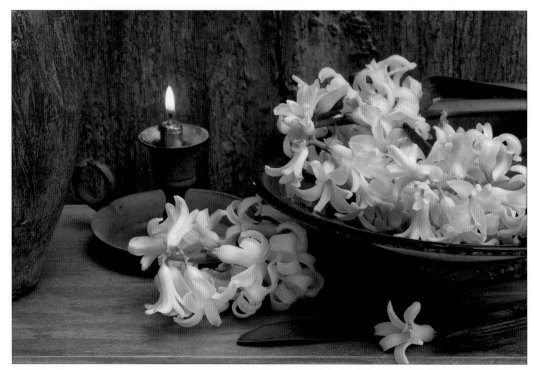

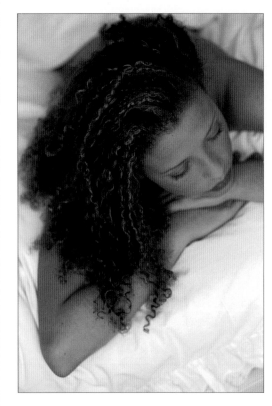

ABOVE: Surrounded by the heady scent of hyacinths and flickering candlelight, you have set the scene for some serious pampering.

LEFT: Relaxing on your bed for 15 minutes can be very refreshing before an evening out.

scented and you are treating yourself to a face pack, your restless body will be held captive and, with any luck, will capitulate and enjoy the experience. Establish your relaxing bath as a regular ritual and encourage your family to respect your privacy: you will all benefit from the calmer, happier person who emerges.

Create your own sanctuary in your bathroom, to where you can retreat to improve your health, pamper your skin or try out some of the beauty routines you would be offered at a professional salon or a health spa. Make yourself comfortable: invest in a blow-up pillow and a bath rack that will hold a book and a glass of wine as well as your bathing essentials. Play soothing music, warm your towels and bathrobe and switch on the answering machine or take the phone off the hook. As you spend more time on yourself, you will become more aware of the needs of your body and how to treat it and soon you will find yourself feeling fitter and looking better.

⤙ BATHED IN FRAGRANCE ⤚

Familiarize yourself with aromatherapy oils and use them for therapeutic baths, for fragrance in your beauty preparations or simply for pure pleasure. A few drops of essential oil in a warm bath can help ease a cold, alleviate insomnia or relieve anxiety. Fragrance has an incredible ability to affect your mood and, once you have experimented with your favourites, you will get to know what to use when you want to sparkle, or feel alluring or tranquil. Enjoy smoothing and scenting your skin with fragrant creams, lotions and powders. These are ancient rituals that women have performed for thousands of years, not solely to make themselves more alluring to others but also to acknowledge and enjoy their femaleness.

forget words like "regime" and "programme", which sound far too much like hard work, and think of softer, more enjoyable concepts such as "cherish" and "pamper". Take yourself off to the bathroom for a session of "serious pampering", which sounds like a lot more fun than carrying out a "rigorous skin-cleansing programme", and yet they can be one and the same thing — it's only the approach and attitude of mind that differs.

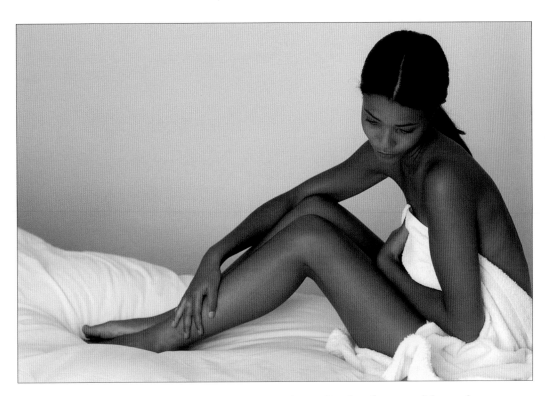

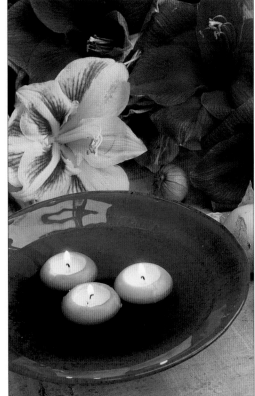

THE HEALING TOUCH

Of all the pleasures to be enjoyed when we take time to care for ourselves, few can rival a soothing massage. In an ideal world, we would all have a daily massage carried out by a caring and patient companion with nothing in mind other than our pleasure. In the real world, it is necessary to compromise and find a way to have our needs met without becoming inconsiderate or resentful.

If time and money permits, a regular professional massage is an incomparable tactile

ABOVE: Regular self massage helps you become familiar with unnecessary muscle tension in your body and deal with it before it causes aches and pains.

RIGHT: Floating candles add a meditative touch.

treat but even self-massage can help you de-stress and relax. In the same way that a regular exercise programme can help tone the body, so regular self-massage can relax tense muscles and promote a feeling of well-being.

When it comes to caring for your skin

Pampering

RELAXATION

~·~

It is essential to find the time to switch off from our daily concerns and find some private time for ourselves. This can be incredibly difficult: we all have so many demands made upon us, whether we are parents of young children, working people or

BELOW: A voluminous bathrobe is the perfect apparel for relaxation.

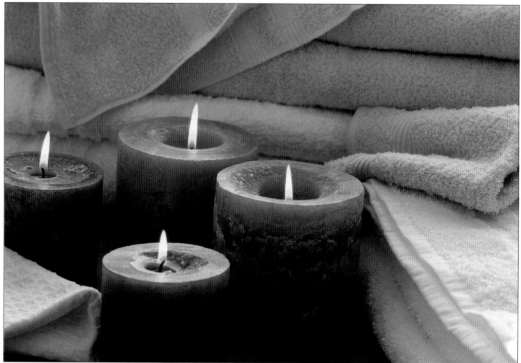

ABOVE: A good supply of clean, fluffy towels and beautiful candles can make taking a bath a glorious indulgence.

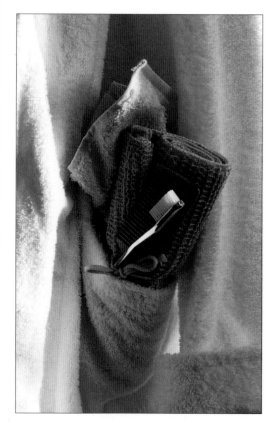

stressed professionals, all of us have far too many calls upon our time and habitually put our own needs last. We get used to self-sacrifice and feel uncomfortable when we put our needs first. We need to retrain ourselves — starting slowly — by simply giving yourself a fresh towel and bathing in water that is scented with a handful of bath salts.

Having established with yourself and the rest of the household that the bathroom is to be your territory for at least half an hour, you can begin to experiment so that you can find

out which of the relaxation techniques you find most beneficial.

Candlelight has a wonderful ability to slow the pace, and when it is combined with warm, scented water, it can turn an ordinary bath into an occasion and leave you far more refreshed than normal. Sometimes, silence is a welcome and a necessary rest from our noisy world, while at other times we need the solace of a favourite piece of music. Be sensitive to your mood and your needs; if your eyes are tired and aching, you would gain more from lying back with some soothing eye compresses than from reading a book, even if reading a book in the bath is your idea of bliss. In other words, the key to successful relaxation is arranging a regular time and place where you will have the opportunity to be alone and using this time to refresh your body and spirit.

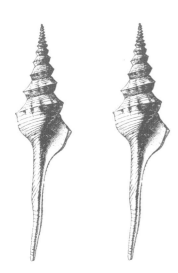

RIGHT: There are times when we all need to let our hair down, relax in a comfortable chair and forget about our everyday life.

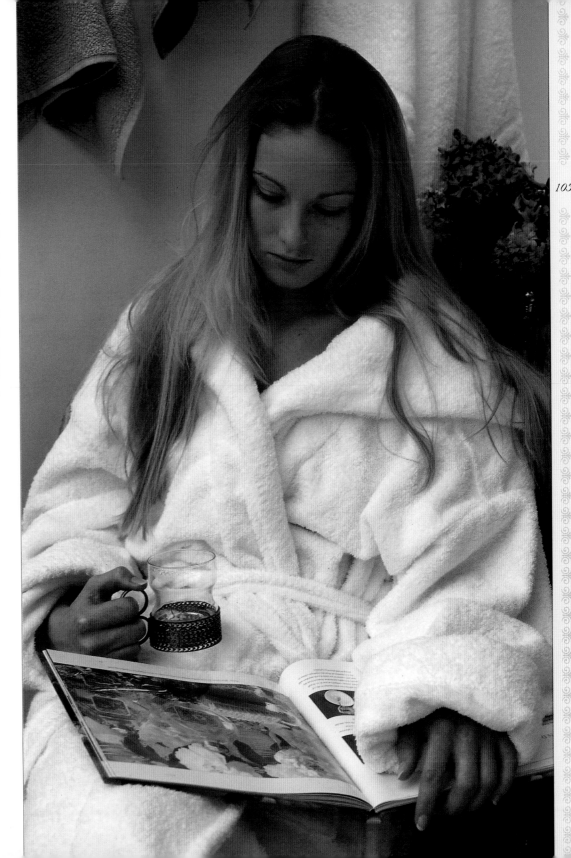

AROMATHERAPY

The term aromatherapy was first coined in the 1920s, although it wasn't really until the 1960s that it became a recognized therapeutic treatment. Since then, aromatherapy has become increasingly popular, both as an effective alternative therapy and a source of useful home remedies as well as a wonderful way to enjoy pure fragrances.

Aromatherapy uses pure essential oils obtained from plants. With very few exceptions, these oils should always be diluted before use, because the pure oils are extremely powerful. Anyone who has an existing medical condition, has very sensitive skin or is pregnant should check before using the oils but, that having been said, one should not be put off because using essential oils is enormously pleasurable.

The cost of the oils varies greatly, depending on the difficulty of extracting them from the plant, so it is sensible to start with some of the less expensive oils and only move on to the more precious oils as you become accustomed to using them.

A good starter collection would consist of lavender, geranium, ti-tree and grapefruit oils and, ideally, would also include chamomile, which, although more expensive, is one of the most useful oils. All these oils are used in projects featured in the previous chapter and will allow you to experiment with them and gain confidence. If you become really enthusiastic about their use, buy a comprehensive guide to aromatherapy, which will give detailed information about the properties of each oil and their appropriate uses.

All essential oils should be stored in a cool place away from the light. You can buy boxes specially made for the purpose, or use a

BELOW: Essential oils should always be stored away from the light in a cool place. This little casket is ideal for the purpose.

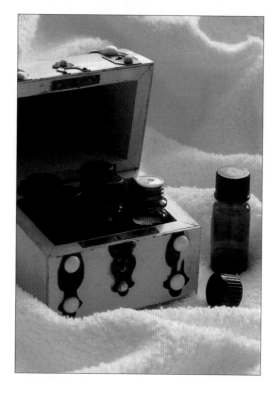

decorative wooden box or even a sturdy cardboard box; however you store them, be sure to keep the oils out of the reach of children. Oils have different shelf lives: the citrus oils, for instance, should be used within six months. Before using, check that the oils still smell fresh, and throw them away if there is any hint of rancidity, as rancid oils can irritate the skin. Some oils need to be used with caution, and details of where this applies to the oils used in this book appear in the section The Safe Use of Natural Products.

Essential oils for massages and for adding to baths should be mixed with a number of different base oils, as the oils undiluted would be far too strong to apply to the skin. Almond oil is generally considered to be one of the mildest and least likely to cause any skin irritation, but there are a number of different oils that are also very pleasant to use, such as jojoba, avocado or grapeseed oil. To be quite sure that the oil is safe to use, you should carry out a patch test on a small area of your skin.

The use of essential oils is not limited to therapeutic and cosmetic purposes; they can also be used to scent the air and to add extra fragrance to pot-pourris, and some of them may also be used in cooking.

You can disperse their fragrance in a room in various ways, by simply adding a couple of

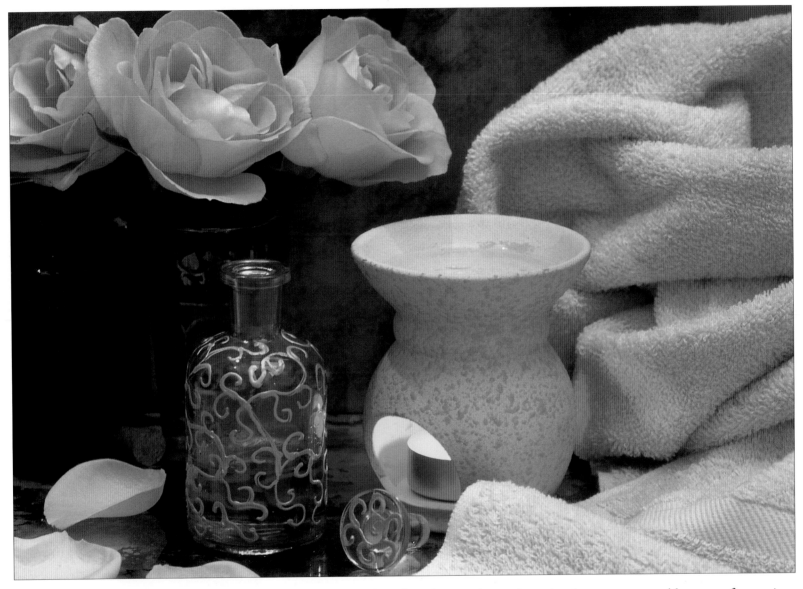

drops of your chosen oil to the melted pool of wax around the wick of a burning candle, by diluting the oil with water and spraying the air from an aerosol bottle, or by vaporizing the oil in a burner or on a light-bulb ring made specially for the purpose. The burners are usually ceramic (although you can also use

ABOVE: Essential oils can be used to scent the room by mixing them with water and vaporizing them in a specially made burner.

terracotta ones, glazed on the inside) and consist of a shallow bowl above a pierced container that holds a night-light. When vaporizing oils

in a burner, pour a tablespoon of water into the shallow dish and add a few drops of oil. Alternatively, drip a couple of drops of neat oil on to the light-bulb ring and then put it over the top of the bulb; it will quickly diffuse the aroma into the surrounding air. Don't leave burners unattended when lit.

SCENTS AND PERFUMES

The power of fragrance to influence and alter moods and behaviour has been understood for thousands of years and continues to be central to our lives, although we may not always realize it. Practically every household product and sometimes even the air we breathe in large buildings has been given a particular fragrance by industrial chemists, who understand that different fragrances have different effects. Lemon and pine give the impression of freshness and cleanliness and

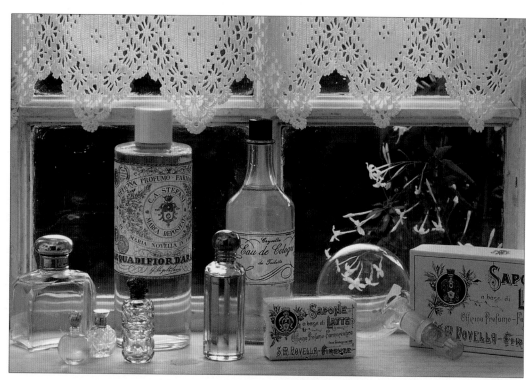

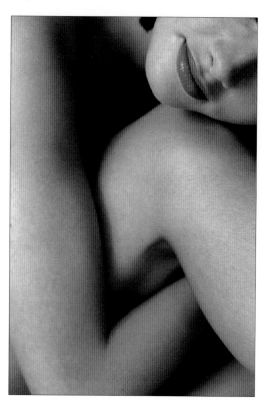

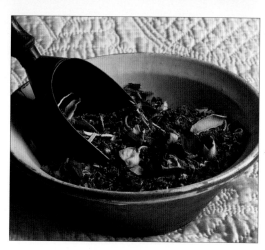

ABOVE: Old scent bottles make a lovely display in a window, but they should be filled with coloured water, rather than scent, as it deteriorates quickly in the light.

LEFT: Scent should be applied to the pulse points, behind the knees and inside the elbows rather than just sprayed around the throat.

RIGHT: Pot-pourri is a subtle and attractive way to scent a room. If the smell fades away you can refresh the bowl with a few drops of essential oil.

peppermint is invigorating, while lavender is nostalgic. Just as they use fragrance to create a certain mood and sell their products, so we can use scent and perfume to suit our personality and enhance our lives.

It is generally accepted that the best way to use a scent on the body is to "layer" it, by using a variety of scented products rather than

BELOW: A wire soap dish featuring a heart design is the perfect container for the soaps, which look as if they were made to go with it.

simply spraying yourself with your chosen fragrance. So, a bath oil, soap, dusting powder, body lotion and *eau de toilette* will each add a layer of fragrance, some of which will, fairly rapidly, evaporate into the air, while others will be absorbed into the skin and release the fragrance over many hours.

A favourite blend of essential oils can be used in the making of the full range of soaps, oils, creams and powders, to allow you to build up subtle layers of your favourite fragrance. Like essential oils, scents and perfumes

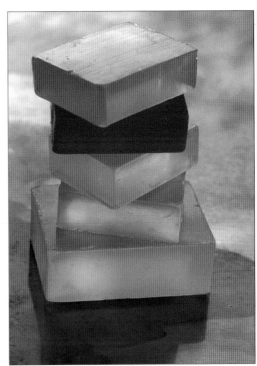

BELOW: Clear glycerine soaps in fruit gum colours look almost good enough to eat.

should be stored away from the light in a fairly cool position. As pretty as all those bottles may look on your dressing table, the fragrances will soon deteriorate unless given some protection. You should keep commercially produced scents and perfumes in their box, while home-made fragrances are best stored in coloured glass bottles out of the light. The pretty bottles on the dressing table can always be filled with coloured water!

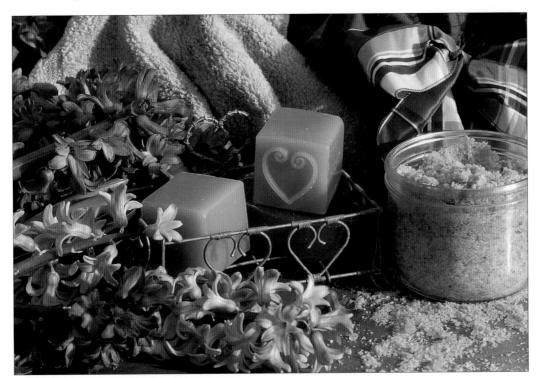

MASSAGE

Anyone will benefit from regular massage from a qualified masseur or masseuse, whose skilled ministrations will not only ease tense muscles but also help us feel warm and relaxed.

Although quite different and inevitably limited, self-massage is also an excellent way to help yourself relax and can help clear tension headaches and ease a stiff neck and shoulders.

Once again, the benefit is not only from the gentle application of massage oil but also from the time taken to care for yourself and your needs. These techniques can be used to give relief from cramped muscles wherever you are but, ideally, should be carried out just before a bath or when you can lie down in a warm place.

Prepare for self-massage in the same way as you would if you were massaging another person: play some soft music, lower the lighting or light candles, make sure the room is warm, that any clothes you are wearing are loose, and that you are sitting in a comfortable position on a chair or on the floor with a clean towel spread beneath you.

The oil for the massage, blended with essential oil, should be poured into a small, clean bowl from where you can take more oil from time to time without disturbing the rhythm of the massage. Stand the bowl of oil on a towel to protect the surface.

RELIEVING NECK TENSION

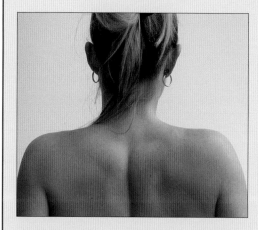

1 Shrug your shoulders and at the same time push them back as far as possible, hold for a count of 5 and then relax completely. Repeat 5 times.

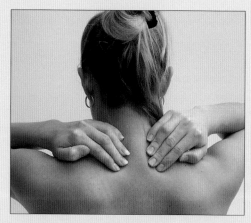

3 Press the back of your neck with the fingers of both hands and move your fingertips in an outward circular motion. Start at your shoulders and work up to the base of the skull. Repeat 5 times.

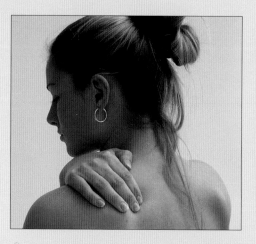

2 Starting at the top of your arm, knead firmly, moving slowly towards your neck. Repeat the movements in the opposite direction back to the edge of your shoulder. Repeat three times on either side.

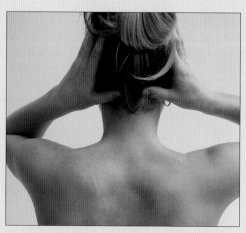

4 Gently hold your head and position your thumbs so that they are at the base of the skull. Rotate your thumbs, using moderate pressure. Do ten rotations, rest your arms and then repeat twice more.

FACE MASSAGE

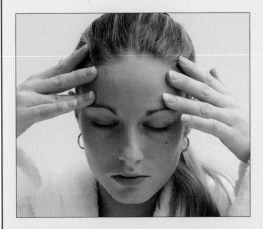

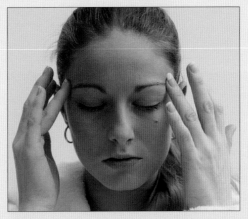

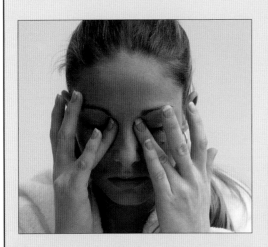

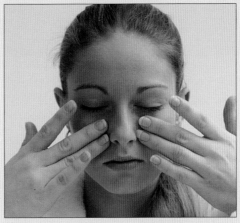

1 Starting in the centre of your forehead, make small circular motions with your fingertips and work slowly outwards towards the temples. Repeat 3 times.

3 Move your fingers outwards along the brow bone from the top of your nose. Repeat 5 times.

2 Use your fingers to gently apply pressure to the area where the eye socket meets your nose. Repeat 3 times.

4 Starting either side of your nose, move your fingers outwards using circular motions along the cheekbone to the jaw. Pay particular attention to the jaw area. Repeat 5 times.

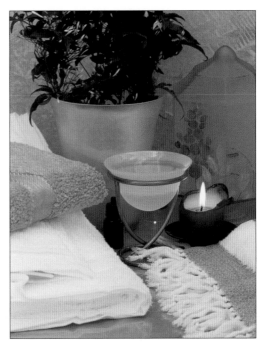

ABOVE: When preparing for a massage be sure to have everything you need at hand. It is distracting to have to break off half way through to replenish the oil or fetch a warm towel.

Choose the blend of oils for the massage according to your needs: if you are tense and overtired, a relaxing blend of lavender, which is good for easing tension headaches, chamomile and clary sage could be helpful; if you need revitalizing, geranium and bergamot will give you a lift and, if you are planning a romantic evening with your partner, get yourself in the mood with rose or jasmine.

There is an undoubted sensuality about massage, the feel of oil on the skin and the gradual easing of tension, so enjoy this opportunity to pamper yourself.

CLEANSING AND MOISTURIZING

A regular routine of cleansing and moisturizing the skin will keep it looking its best, no matter what your age. The choice of cleanser is really a matter of personal preference: there are those who feel that their skin is never really clean unless it has been washed, while others throw up their hands in horror at the thought of water coming anywhere near the face. Both methods are effective and neither is superior to the other, provided that the

BELOW: Exfoliating the skin removes dead skin cells and leaves the skin looking clean and healthy.

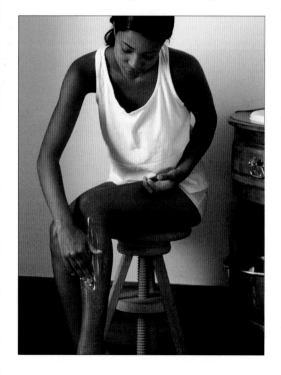

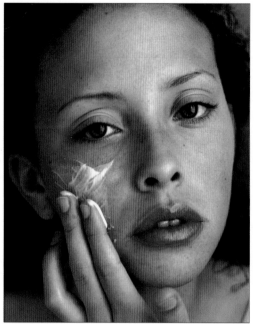

ABOVE: Cream cleansers gently lift dirt and make-up from the face and are ideal for dry skins.

products you use are made from pure ingredients and are not harsh upon the skin.

Cleansers which use water are usually creams or bars that you liquefy in the palm with water and gently rub over your face before splashing off with lukewarm water. Soapwort cleanse is used in this way and is particularly suitable for those with very sensitive skins. After cleansing in this way, the skin both looks and feels toned and refreshed.

Cream cleansers are gently massaged into the skin and then wiped off with moist cotton wool, taking with the cream any remnants of make-up, dead skin and dirt. For thorough cleansing, a second application of cream will ensure that the skin is thoroughly cleaned. Cleansing with a cream cleanser leaves the skin feeling soft and supple.

Before moisturizing, it is advisable for those with oily skin or enlarged pores to splash the face with cold water or use an astringent tonic.

Only use moisturizer on thoroughly cleaned skin or you will be trapping impurities, which can cause spots and skin irritation. Dab the moisturizer on to your forehead, cheeks, chin and nose and neck and then gently massage it into the skin, using delicate

BELOW: Oily skins can benefit from the use of a cleansing bar used with water and applied with a soft facial sponge.

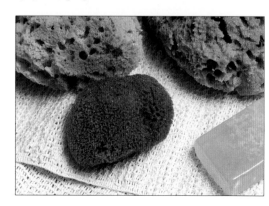

upward strokes, and pat it in around the tender eye area. If your skin is feeling particularly parched, cleanse it thoroughly then apply a liberal coat of moisturizing cream. Lie back in the bath and allow the skin to absorb the cream before dabbing away any excess by placing an opened tissue over your face.

RIGHT: Your moisturizing cream should leave your skin feeling soft and smooth.

BELOW: Always treat the area round the eyes very carefully, applying creams with a dabbing motion.

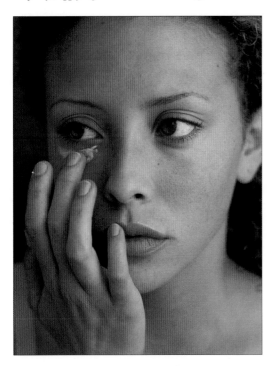

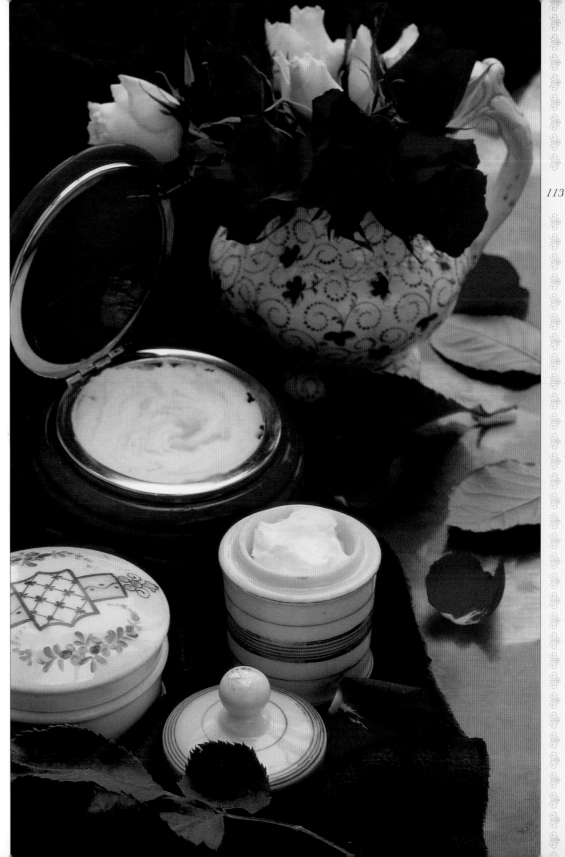

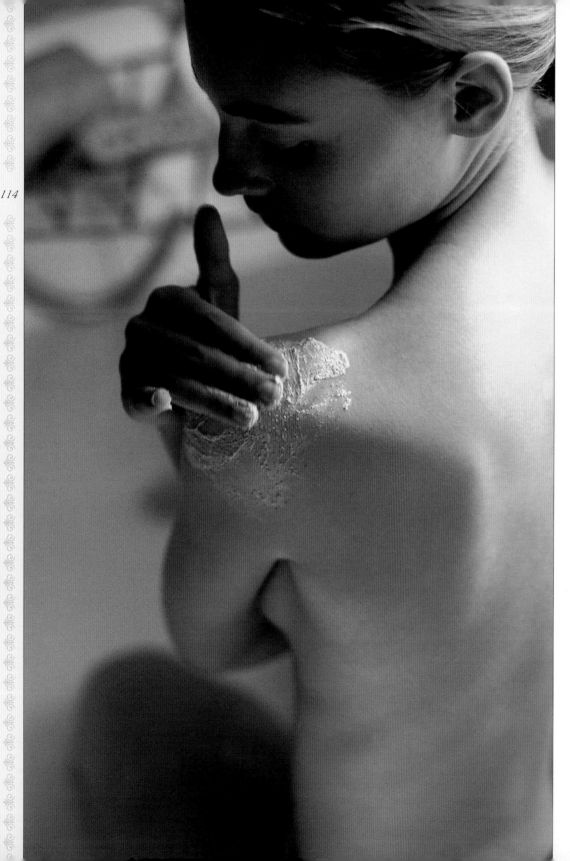

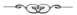

Pampering

BODY SCRUBS

*I*n the absence of water, women of the Middle East would coat their skin with perfumed oil and then rub themselves clean with handfuls of sand, so, although the use of body scrubs is comparatively new to the West, it has a long and honourable tradition as a way of promoting good circulation and a glowing, healthy skin.

Modern body scrubs generally consist of a blend of ingredients, some of which will gently remove dead skin and ingrained dirt while others soften and nourish the skin. Every cosmetic house will have a selection to sell you but, as this is one of the easiest and least expensive to make at home, you may prefer to follow the recipe for Citrus Body Scrub.

Before you start you will need to mix 3 tablespoons of the scrub to a stiff paste with almond oil. The scrub is then ready to use. You will find an empty bath by far the most convenient place to use an exfoliator.

Remove all your clothes and stand in the bath or sit on a folded towel on the side. Starting with your shoulders and arms, smear the paste on your skin and gently work it over the surface, using a circular motion and paying particular attention to any areas of rough skin; avoid tender skin, bruises or cuts. Work

LEFT: Body scrubs are not a new idea; ancient civilizations have used them for thousands of years.

FACE SCRUB

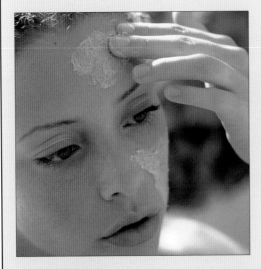

1 Gently massage the scrub into the face and neck using circular movements, taking care to avoid the eye area.

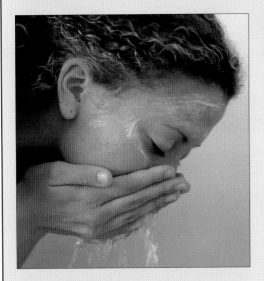

2 Splash the face with lukewarm water until all traces of the scrub are removed and pat dry with a clean towel.

BODY SCRUB

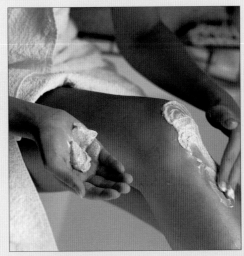

1 To exfoliate the legs, mix the scrub with water to make a paste and work into the skin using firm finger pressure.

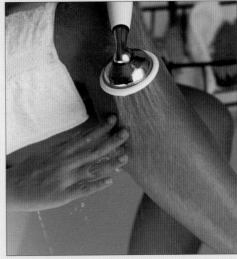

2 Use a dry flannel to remove most of the scrub and then rinse the remnants away with cold water.

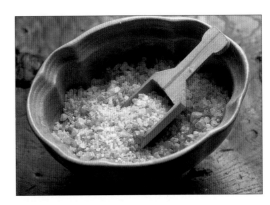

ABOVE: Coarse sea salt can be used in the bath and can also be included in body scrubs to assist exfoliation.

your way down your body until you reach the knees, ankles and feet, which will all benefit from extra attention. To finish, rub over the body with a clean, dry flannel to remove any scrub which still adheres to the body and to stimulate your circulation. Shower or bathe as usual. You will emerge from the bath with glowing skin and a feel of healthy well-being.

For the delicate skin of the face, choose a fine-textured scrub and use it in gentle, circular massaging movements all over the face and neck, avoiding the delicate eye area.

Loofahs, sponges and sisal cloths can also be used to exfoliate and improve skin tone, but do be careful not to use these too vigorously or they can damage the skin. Use them on wet skin and only on less sensitive areas of the body and take care not to damage moles.

HANDS AND FEET

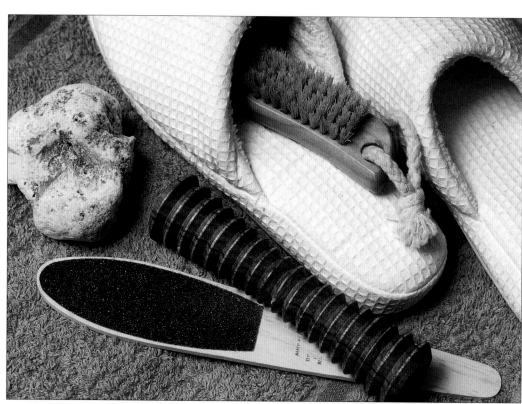

116 ℘ositioned at the extremities of our bodies, our hands and feet are essential equipment that we tend to take very much for granted – until something goes wrong. Like a regularly serviced car, hands and feet will prove far more reliable in the long run if we take a little time to look after them.

Investing in a basic manicure set is a good start and, with the addition of emery boards, a pumice stone, a nail-brush and nourishing creams, you will have all you need to keep hands and feet in tip-top condition.

Keep your manicure set in the bathroom so that you can attend to your hands and feet while you are lying in the bath. The water softens the skin and the nails and makes them easier to work on. Firstly, brush the nails thoroughly with the nail-brush and attend to any hard skin with the pumice stone before cutting and shaping the nails. Moisturize the

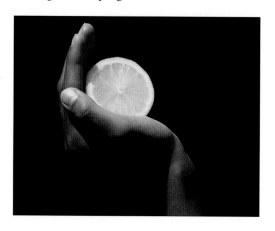

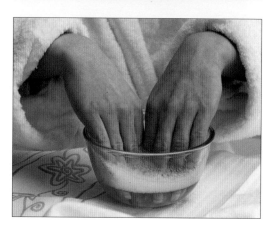

ABOVE: Investing in a few pieces of equipment, such as a pumice stone and rough skin remover, will allow you to keep your feet in excellent condition.

LEFT: Lemon juice is a useful natural skin softener and cleanser for neglected hands.

RIGHT: Soak your fingernails in a bowl of warm, soapy water before giving yourself a manicure. Use a gentle, unscented soap, not a harsh detergent.

hands and feet, along with the rest of the body, when you leave the bath, or use a richer formula for particularly dry skin.

Keep a bottle of hand cream next to the kitchen sink and use it whenever you finish washing up; have another bottle next to the bed to apply before you sleep. For emergency treatment for very cracked and uncomfortable skin, apply the cream thickly and then sleep in a pair of cotton gloves.

RIGHT AND BELOW: Feet are often neglected but will benefit hugely from some care and attention.

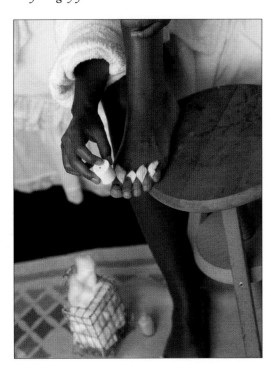

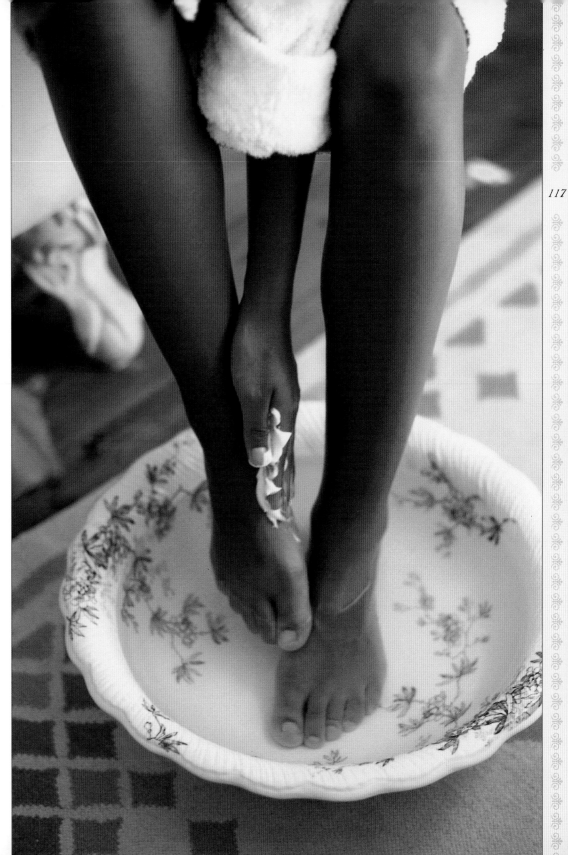

FACIALS

As well as the daily cleansing and mois-turizing routines, it is good to programme in time for a facial at least once a month. This is another opportunity to take yourself off to the bathroom, lock the door and indulge in some serious facial care.

There are a number of treatments that will improve the texture and condition of your skin, and you can alternate these until you find the treatment that best suits your skin.

BELOW: Don't neglect your neck when giving yourself a facial. Use gentle upward movements.

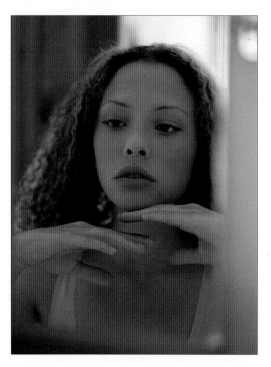

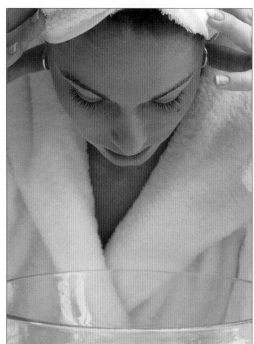

ABOVE: Steaming your face will help cleanse the skin by opening the pores.

You will gain maximum benefit from all these treatments if you carry them out at time when you do not need to apply make-up afterwards: ideally, just before you go to bed.

STEAMING

To steam your face, wrap your hair in a towel and hold your head over a bowl of hot, steam-ing water. You could scent the water with a couple of drops of a favourite essential oil.

An oil which is good for skin would be ther-apeutic as well as pleasant – lavender, rose, frankincense and sandalwood all have this quality. For a sauna effect, drape another towel over your head and the bowl, so that the steam is trapped and the steaming effect intensified. The steam will open pores and cleanse the skin. Ten minutes of steaming should be fol-lowed by splashing the face with cold water, which will wash away the residues and tighten

BELOW: It is important to moisturize your skin after a facial, but let it rest for a few minutes before doing so.

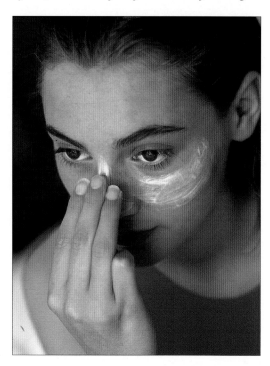

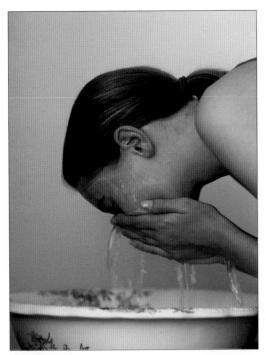

ABOVE: *After massaging it into the skin, splash away a facial scrub with plenty of lukewarm water.*

the pores. Rest the face for a few minutes before applying a moisturizer.

⊸ FACIAL SCRUBS ⊶

These would be better called "facial rubs", as the last thing that you should do to your face is scrub it. These scrubs are similar to, but more gentle in action than, the body scrubs. If you are using the gentle face scrub from this book, you will need to mix the scrub into a smooth paste with almond oil. Gently smear the scrub on to your face, avoiding the delicate area around the eyes. Use small, circular movements to lift and loosen the dead skin cells on the surface of the skin. Use lukewarm water to wash the scrub from your skin and

pat your face dry with a clean, soft towel. Leave the face to rest for at least 5 minutes before applying moisturizer.

⊸ FACE MASKS ⊶

Ideally, you should apply a face mask after you have given your skin a deep cleansing by steaming or gentle exfoliation, but, in either case, it is wise to rest the skin for at least 10 minutes before applying the mask or the skin may be overstimulated and have a sensitive reaction.

There are an enormous range of face masks on the market to suit every skin type, from very oily to very dry. Spend time choosing a formulation which suits your skin and always do a patch test first, to ensure that it does not cause sensitivity. The 2 recipes given for face masks in this book are both suitable for most skin types, but those with extremely sensitive skins should avoid any face masks that contain clays.

Before embarking on a face mask, make certain that you will be able to have an uninterrupted half hour. Switch on the answering machine and tell the family that you are not to be disturbed – this is not just because you will look somewhat tribal daubed with face mask but also to ensure that they won't be asking you questions through the bathroom door – a face mask is most effective when you

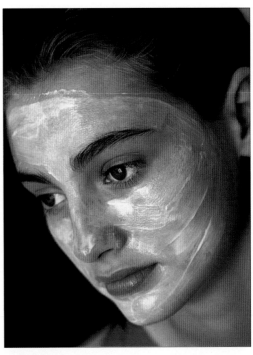

ABOVE: *Sit quietly while your face mask works its magic. This is not the time for an animated conversation.*

can keep your face immobile for 15 minutes. As this is an ideal opportunity to relax, run a nice deep bath ready for you to climb into once you have applied the face mask. If you have time, give your face a steam facial or an exfoliation treatment first; if not, cleanse the skin thoroughly and then smooth the face mask over the face, avoiding the delicate skin around the eyes and mouth. Lie back and relax and let the face mask work its magic. After 15 minutes, wash the face mask off with lukewarm water and then splash your face with cold water before patting dry with a clean towel. Wait for 5 minutes before applying moisturizer. A weekly face mask will keep your skin in wonderful condition.

120

Many people wash their hair daily these days and there are myriad shampoos that allow us to do this without stripping the hair of its oils. Hair-care experts also recommend that you should change your shampoo every now and again or, better still, alternate between two different ones, to keep your hair looking its best.

In spite of what the advertisements may tell us, we do not need to condition our hair every day – for normal hair, once a week will do; for dry hair, three times a week is sufficient. The problem with over-conditioning your hair is that the conditioner can build up on your hair and scalp and lead to dull, lifeless hair, just the reverse of what you are hoping to achieve. The two-in-one shampoos and conditioners are particularly prone to do this and should be avoided.

BELOW: Healthy, well-cared for hair is a joy for others to look at and makes you feel wonderful.

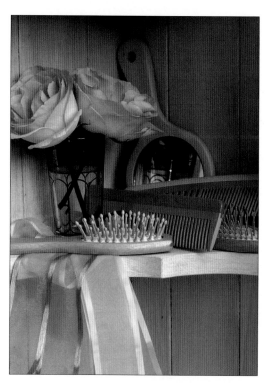

ABOVE: Your hair will benefit from good quality brushes and combs that are kept clean.

─◌ HERBAL HAIR RINSES ◌─

Aside from regular shampooing, there are a number of home treatments which will promote hair and scalp health and help to avoid any build up of shampoo residues in your hair. Alternate using a cream conditioner on your hair with one of the herbal rinses in the previous chapter. These will leave your hair feeling squeaky-clean and looking glossy.

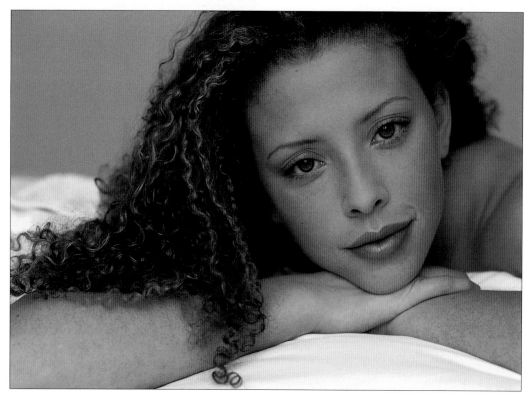

Simply replace the last water rinse with a jugful of the herbal rinse, mixed 50/50 with water, and leave it to dry.

⟶ INTENSIVE HAIR TREATMENTS ⟵
Regular deep-conditioning of the hair will help to promote glossy, lustrous hair. Most shampoo manufacturers now offer this type of treatment in their range, usually in two formulas, cream-based and oil-based. Recipes for home-made versions appear in the previous chapter. Use the cream-based treatments after shampooing; comb them gently through damp hair, leave on the hair to be absorbed for 5–20 minutes and then rinse off with warm, but not hot, water.

Use the oil treatments on dry hair before shampooing. Carefully work the oil into the hair and scalp, which should be coated all the way through without being saturated. Gently comb through the hair, to make sure every strand is coated, and then wrap the hair in a hot towel for 20 minutes. Use a gentle shampoo as normal but do not condition.

HAIR TREATMENT

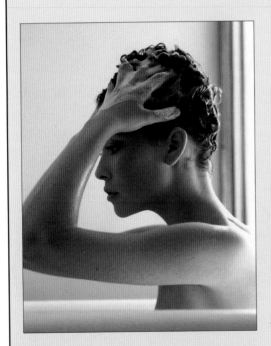

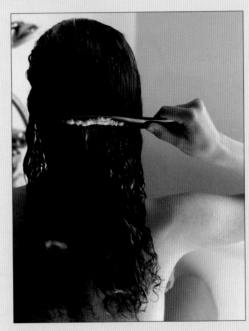

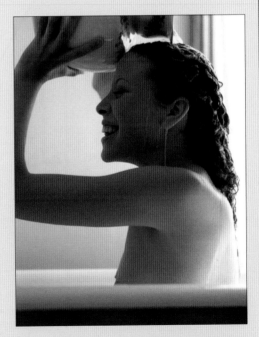

1 Hair washing is also an opportunity for gentle scalp massage; gently work all over your scalp using circular movements.

2 Smooth cream conditioner over the hair and then comb it through to ensure it coats the hair evenly.

3 A final rinse of cool water may make you shudder temporarily but will leave your scalp tingling and refreshed.

TEMPLATES

To enlarge the templates, use either a grid system or a photocopier. For the grid system, trace the template and draw a grid of evenly spaced squares over the tracing. To scale up, draw a larger grid on to another piece of paper. Copy the outline on to the second grid by taking each square individually and drawing the relevant part of the outline in the larger square. Draw over the lines to make sure they are continuous.

JAUNTY TOWELS
page 56

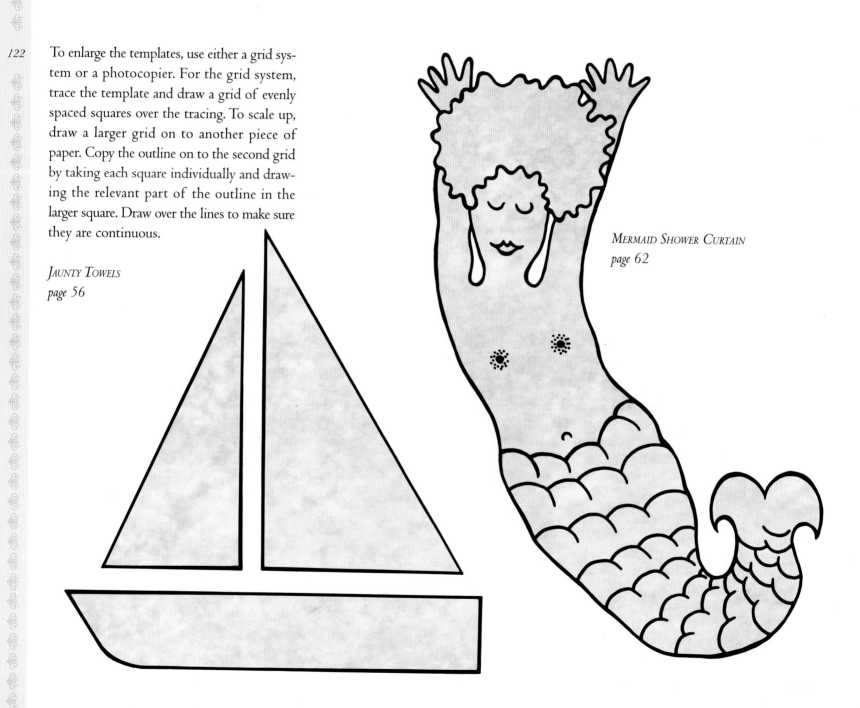

MERMAID SHOWER CURTAIN
page 62

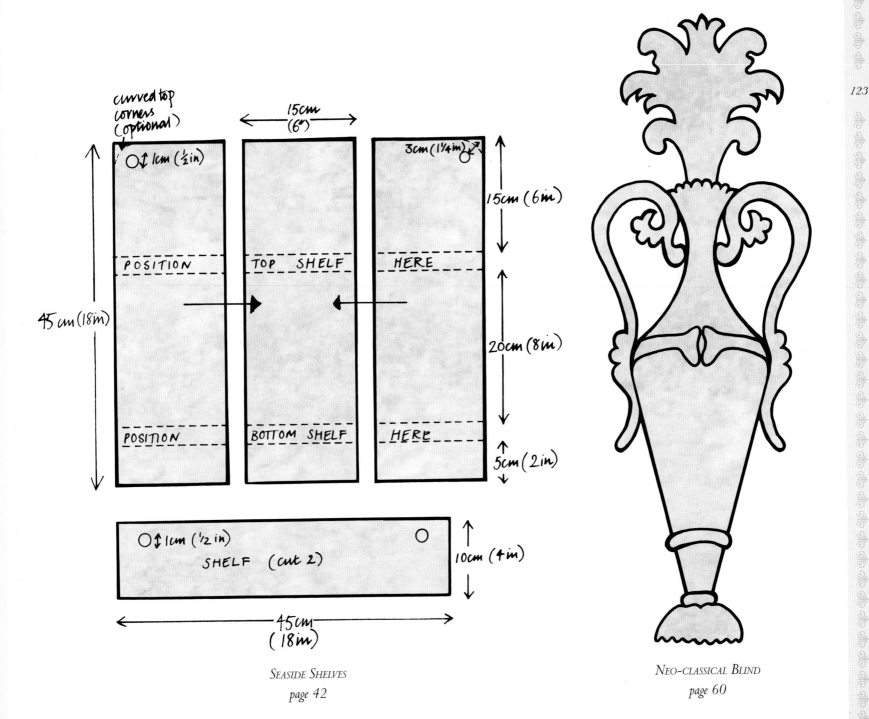

curved top corners (optional)

○↕ 1cm (½in)

15cm (6")

3cm (1¼in)

15cm (6in)

POSITION   TOP   SHELF   HERE

45 cm (18in)

20cm (8in)

POSITION   BOTTOM SHELF   HERE

5cm (2in)

○↕ 1cm (½in)   ○

SHELF   (cut 2)

10cm (4in)

45cm (18in)

SEASIDE SHELVES
page 42

NEO-CLASSICAL BLIND
page 60

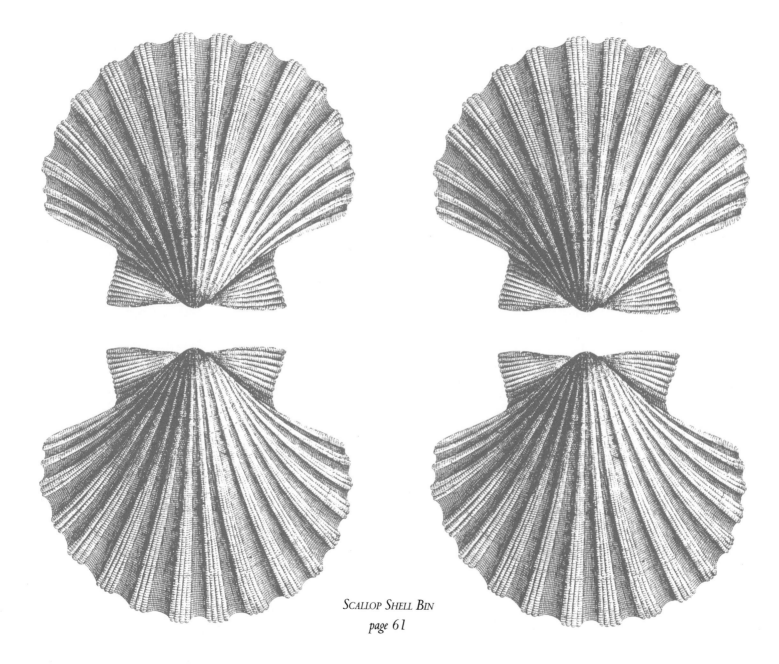

Scallop Shell Bin
page 61

CANDLE-MAKING EQUIPMENT AND MATERIALS:

Candle Maker's Supplies
28 Blythe Road
London W14 0HA
Tel: 0171 602 4031

Dadant & Sons
51 South Second Street
Hamilton, IL 62341
USA
Tel: (217) 847-3324

John L. Guilfoyle Pty Ltd
772 Boundary Road
Darra, Qld 4076
Australia
Tel: (07) 3375 3677

ESSENTIAL OILS:

Fleur Aromatherapy
Pembroke Studios
Pembroke Road
London N10 2JE
Tel: 0181 444 7424

Neal's Yard Remedies
5 Golden Cross
Cornmarket Street
Oxford OX1 3EU
Tel: 01865 245436 for mail-order
catalogue

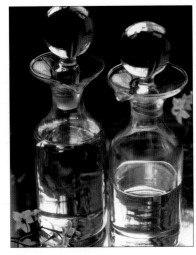

Meadow Everlastings
16464 Shabbona Road
Malta, IL 60150
USA
Tel: (815) 825-2539

Aromatic Products
P.O. Box 840
Southport Business Centre
Southport, Qld 4215
Australia
Tel: (07) 5591 5859

ORGANIC DRIED HERBS, BEESWAX AND PURE ROSE WATER:

Hambleden Herbs
Court Farm
Milverton
Somerset TA4 1NF
Tel: 01823 401205

Shaw Mudge and Co.
P.O. Box 1375
Stamford, CT 06904
USA
Tel: (203) 327-3132

The Craft Company
Corner Victoria Avenue and
Neridah Street
Chatswood, NSW 2067
Australia
Tel: (02) 9413 1781

NATURAL BEAUTY INGREDIENTS:

G. Baldwin and Co.
173 Walworth Road
London SE17 1RW
Tel: 0171 703 5550

Tom Thumb Workshops
P.O. Box 357
Mappsville, VA 23487
USA
Tel: (804) 824-3507

Potions & Lotions
P.O. Box 339
Doubleday Bay, NSW 2028
Australia
Tel: (02) 9314 2268

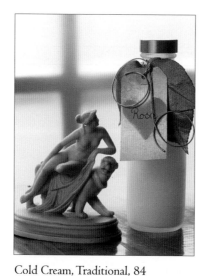
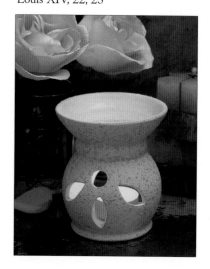

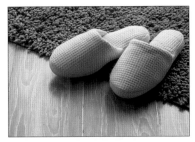

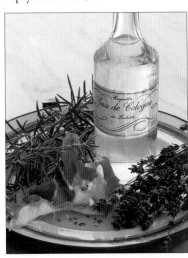

ACKNOWLEDGEMENTS

The publishers would like to thank the following people for the use of their pictures.

The Water Monopoly, 16/18 Lonsdale Road, London, NW6 6RD pp 30, 33, 34, 35, 66.
Simon Bottomley pp 101r, 102l, 103l.

The Bridgeman Art Library: pp 10 *The Bathers* by PA Laurens, Roy Miles Gallery, London; 11l *The Danaides* by John William Waterhouse, Christie's, London; 11r *The Kiss* by Sir Lawrence Alma-Tadema, The Maas Gallery, London; 12l *Anthony and Cleopatra* by Sir Lawrence Alma-Tadema, Private Collection; 13 *The New Perfume* by John William Godward, Christie's, London; 14m *The Bracelet* by Frederic Leighton, The Fine Art Society, London; 15r *Strigils and Sponges* by Sir Lawrence Alma-Tadema; 16 *The Turkish Bath* by Serkis Diranian, Roubaix Museum, France; 19r *The Baths of Caracalla* by Sir Lawrence Alma-Tadema, Private Collection; 22 *The Baths of Pozzuoli* by Girolamo Macchietti, Palazzo Vecchio, Florence; 23l *Louis XIV in his Coronation Robes* by Hyacinthe Rigaud, Louvre, Paris; 23r *The Moorish Bath* by Jean Leon Gerome, Christie's Images; 24 *Woman in her Bath Washing her Leg with Sponge* by Edgar Dégas, Musee d'Orsay, Paris; 25t *The Bath* engraving by Nicolas François Regnault after Pierre Antoine Baudouin, Stapleton Collection; 25b *The Pump Room, Bath* by John Claude Nattes, Victoria Art Gallery, Bath; 26t *John Baptising Jesus* by Archbishop Chichele's Breviary, Lambeth Palace Library, London; 27b *Benares: Bathing Scene at a Ghat on the Ganges* by William Daniells, Victoria and Albert Museum, London.

The Visual Arts Library: pp 9r *Susannah at her Bath* by Altdorfer; 12r *Picture from the Tomb of the Nobles*, Luxor, Egypt; 14l Roman Vase; 14r *Mary, Villa of Mysteries*, Pompeii; 15l *Women Washing*, Museum of Archeology, Bari; 17 *The Toilet of Venus*, Fontainebleau School, Louvre, Paris; 18 *The Tepidarium* by Theodore Chasseriau, Musee d'Orsay, Paris; 19l Vase, Chiusi Museum; 20l *The Bath*, Musee de Cluny, Paris; 20r *The Bath* by Jost Amman; 21t *Massage* by Debat-Ponsant, Museum of Toulouse; 21b *The Bathroom* by Virgil Solis; 26b *Baptism* by Julius Stewart, Los Angeles County Museum of Art; 27t *Japanese Bathroom*; 100 *The Gothic Bathroom* by Jean-Baptiste Mallet, Municipal Museum of Dieppe, France; 101l *Eau de Lubin* by E Grasset.
(r = right, l = left, b = bottom, t = top, m = middle)

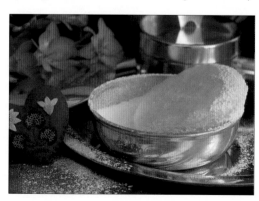

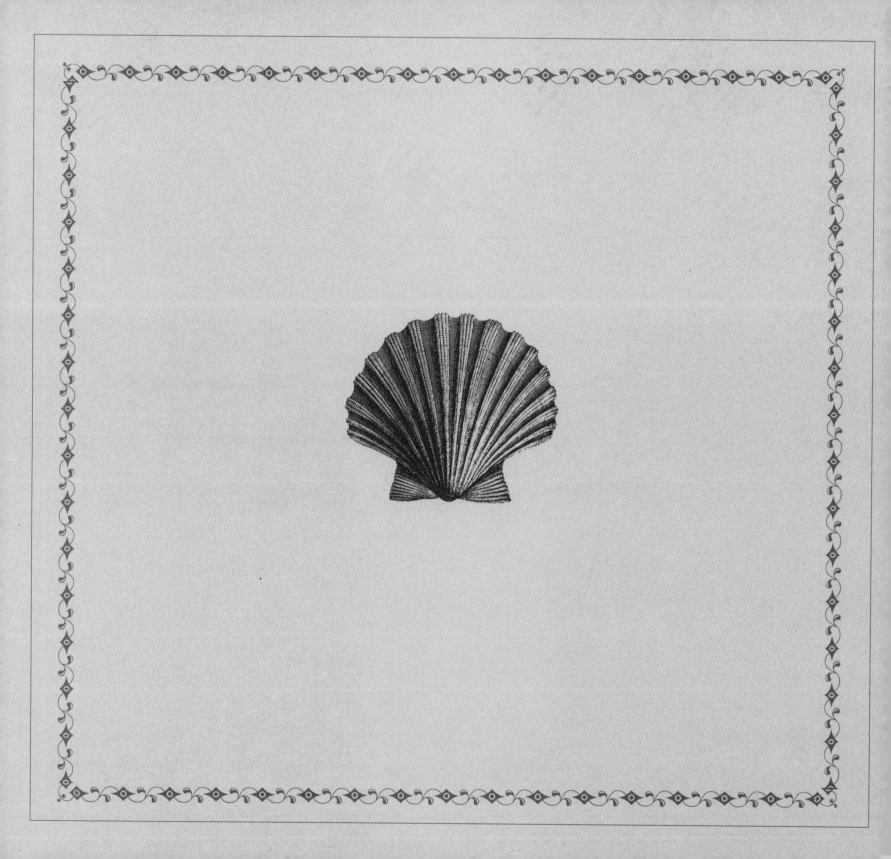